# Video in Mental Health Practice

## An Activities Handbook

## Ira Heilveil

Tavistock Publications

London and New York

First published in Great Britain in 1984 by
Tavistock Publications Ltd
11 New Fetter Lane, London EC4P 4EE

Published in the USA by
Springer Publishing Company, Inc. New York

© 1983 Springer Publishing Company, Inc.

Printed in Great Britain by
J.W. Arrowsmith Ltd, Bristol

British Library Cataloguing in Publication Data

Heilveil, Ira
Video in mental health practice.
1. Video tape in psychotherapy
I. Title
362.2'0425     RC455.2.A92

ISBN 0-422-78800-7

To my parents

# Contents

## 7. Training and Supervision                                                   **112**

## 8. Special Populations                                                         **144**

## 9. Special Applications/Advanced Technology                        **169**

# Foreword

The author of this handbook has moved us boldly into the second generation of video as an adjunctive tool in the everyday work life of helping professionals. Despite the resistance of many colleagues and some patients, the first generation of pioneers creatively explored the potential of video as a teaching, supervisory, and treatment aid during the three decades preceding publication of this book.

The pioneers persisted in gathering data; they did comparative studies of work with patients and clients who did and who did not experience video self-confrontation. As they worked, they integrated the use of video into all accepted theories, thus opening a path for a new generation of creative colleagues whose work is presented in this volume. The pioneers demonstrated the value of their work year after year in workshops and programs, at meetings of the American Psychiatric Association, the American Group Psychotherapy Association, the Orthopsychiatric Association, and the American Psychological Association. Their contribution has been accepted as an aspect of a holistic, scientific approach toward helping people see and know themselves more truthfully and more thoroughly. Ira Heilveil carries the most important message from the pioneers: Video is not a therapeutic modality in itself, but, rather, it is a facilitative electronic miracle akin to the use of the microscope in the field of biology.

The author clearly lives up to his stated purpose "to provide a practical handbook of how to use video within different therapeutic contexts." Heilveil proposes ways for an individual to come to grips with the differences (as described by Karen Horney) between one's idealized image of oneself and one's actual self presented to and experienced by others. I was particularly pleased with the author's sensitivity to the wide range of individuals " . . . from young children to octogenarians, from the mildly neurotic to the blatantly psychotic . . . " who can benefit from the use of video, as well as to the individuals who would probably be best suited to other adjunctive therapeutic tools.

Heilveil has presented in condensed form not only the imaginative techniques developed by others but also a number of techniques he developed himself. The techniques described run the gamut from those aimed at confronting and undermining psychopathology to those of a purely educative and growth-enhancing nature. Heightening skills in students for job interviews, improving interviewing skills in rehabilitating prison inmates, and expanding communication skills in all the people we see in our professional work—these are some additional benefits to be derived from video.

The author has entitled many video activities in an intriguing fashion. "The Naked Eye," "Transfer, Please", "Speed Shift", and "All That Jazz" are just a few of the many activities included. In one technique in Chapter 3 entitled "Voice-over", the author reveals his particular therapeutic style, his personality, and his theory. The other activities in Chapter 3 also give us an intimate and delightful glimpse of Ira Heilveil at his creative best. The piece on "Video Games" demonstrates how video can be used diagnostically in this era of home television games and how video can build rapport between a therapist and children or adolescents. "Video Art Therapy" and "Movement Therapy" in Chapter 4 offer much stimulation to group therapy trainees by opening them up to group process awareness on levels and dimensions not ordinarily examined. All of the subsequent chapters also present imaginative and practical activities that professionals will find most helpful.

This book offers a comprehensive and exciting presentation of most of the creative applications of video in the daily work of helping professionals. It offers realistic ways to promote health and skills in daily living while undermining resistance to change. I recommend it highly to all helping professionals.

Milton M. Berger, M.D.
New York

# Acknowledgements

I am indebted to the many pioneers in the use of video in psychotherapy and training who had the courage to confront the new and the wisdom to retain what is valuable of the old. Reading their work encouraged me to experiment with their techniques, and to invent some of my own. There are too many of them to list here, but their names are scattered throughout the book and will soon become familiar to the reader.

On a more personal note, I would like to thank Marsha McKeon for her critical reading of the manuscript, her support and patience, and the yellow roses.

# 1

# Introduction

If you are in a helping profession, the chances are good that your clinic, school, or hospital has some sort of video equipment, and the chances are also good that the equipment is locked away in a closet collecting dust. One reason this equipment is sadly underutilized is that few clinicians were ever exposed to its use as a clinical tool in their training. Also, some clinicians feel uncomfortable venturing beyond the confines of traditional modes of conducting therapy, or they are frightened by the myth of needing technical acumen to operate video equipment. It is hoped that this book will help to change these attitudes by exposing helpers to some of the myriad effective uses in which videotape technology can be employed therapeutically.

The use of video has recently enjoyed a tremendous surge of interest in the helping professions, due largely to its decreasing cost and subsequent widespread availability. As more therapists use video in their work, an increasing awareness develops among clinicians as to its enormous potential. There is now a large body of anecdotal and research literature on the topic, much of which indicates that through the use of video "confrontation" or "feedback," people come to learn ways in which others may see them, and in so doing they come to see more clearly the ways in which their behavior affects others. The literature also claims that through the use of video, clients may come to deeper insights about themselves sooner than they would have otherwise, and that attitudes, behavior patterns, and traditional roles can be elucidated and modified. Some authors believe that self-concepts can be clarified and altered as clients move toward an increased awareness of their own identity.

These are grand claims, and along with grand claims comes justifiable criticism. Despite the fact that video makes a substantially greater amount of information available than does audiotape, video playback reduces the information that we might derive from a live interview. Emotion is somewhat flattened by the video image; for example, strong anxiety seen in a client during a live interview may seem less dramatic on a TV screen. This may lead the viewer to misconstrue the intensity of the original experience.

Another criticism, infrequently heard but frequently inferred, is that a camera, TV, and video recorder may be seen as gimmicky ways to avoid the intimacy of the psychotherapeutic relationship. It is important to recognize, however, that while video can be an intrusive gimmick, it can also be a powerful tool that can aid the skilled psychotherapist in achieving therapeutic goals of behavior change, insight, catharsis, and enhanced self-esteem. As with any therapeutic technique, the sensitivity and expertise of the therapist will be the primary determinant of how effective an intervention will be.

Several years ago, an article appeared in *Time* magazine (Adams, 1973) about a new form of therapy called "Videotherapy." The use of this term was included in the article over the objections of both the author (Virginia Adams) and the subject (Milton Berger). Since that time, there have been articles written about "Media Therapy" (see Ivey, 1973), and "Teletherapy" (see Brooks, 1976). These names give the false impression that video feedback is a therapeutic modality unto itself, as opposed to being a technique to be used along with other techniques within a therapist's armamentarium.

Video itself is nothing more than a technology. As such it cannot heal. As a tool in the hands of a skilled therapist it can facilitate change, but the factors involved in creating a therapeutic experience—nurturing the seed of hope, the client's internalization of the therapist's positive qualities, learning new habits, insight, catharsis, the empathy of the therapist, genuineness, and so on—are factors which are primarily determined by the relationship between the therapist and the client. As Berger (1978) has pointed out,

> The media is not the therapy or the psychotherapist but rather a facilitative electronic tool similar to what a microscope is to a physician who can better and more appropriately diagnose, prescribe and function as a healer after integrating the data obtained through the medium of the microscope. (p. 138)

It is, however, a flexible and capacious tool, and in the hands of a skilled therapist or teacher, it can be a very valuable therapeutic adjunct.

## General Considerations

Video techniques may be introduced at any point in the therapeutic process, either at the outset or at a particular juncture at which time it may seem useful. While the ways in which video can be applied within therapy are limited only by the imaginations of those using it, there are chiefly two technical approaches to the process. A simultaneous image may be "fed back" by using a television set as a monitor or screen, showing what is being photographed by the camera as it is occurring at the moment; this is the closest the video comes to being a "mirror." The most common use of video in therapy, however, is when a recording, made of a session or part of a session, is played back at a later time for purposes of discussion. It is the choice of the therapist whether to replay a particular set of behaviors in order to highlight them for discussion, or to play back a whole session. Videotapes can be edited in order to present specific moments of significance or interest.

Before embarking on any use of video, it is necessary to obtain permission to videotape the client. The client should be told whether or not tapes made will be used for any purposes other than therapy. If so, it is important to obtain special permission, in written form, for use of the tapes for training or other professional purposes. In most cases, it is a good idea to erase the tapes when they are no longer needed for therapeutic purposes, and the client of course should be informed of this.

Although it may be obvious, it is important to point out the importance of having the video equipment completely visible to the client. The temptation to avoid confrontation with the equipment is strong for those unaccustomed to its use, but any covert use of video techniques will lead to distrust and will subvert long-term goals. The presence of the equipment, while probably the cause of some initial anxiety, decreases significantly after a short time, and in the long run will not hinder the client's trust in the therapist.

Video can be used effectively in individual therapy with children and adults, in group and family therapy, and in the therapeutic classroom. As you will read in the following chapters, videotape feedback has been used creatively in the treatment of a wide variety of difficulties, including behavior disorders, hyperactivity, low self-esteem, alcoholism, drug addiction, depression, sexual dysfunction, and anorexia.

The purpose of this book is to provide a practical handbook of how to use video within different therapeutic contexts. Limitations of its use and considerations for its use within a specific context are discussed in the overviews at the beginning of each chapter.

## Why Does Video Work?

Watching clients watch themselves on video is a remarkable experience. The image on the screen interprets, questions, clarifies, suggests, criticizes, encourages, and contradicts the viewer. Video feedback is a form of self-confrontation, and as such, it asks the client to come face to face with the way in which he or she is seen by the world.

The image presented through video feedback is difficult to dispute. It is a consensually valid mirror, a stark, glaring reality which, in its objectivity, permits a certain emotional distance to form between one's perception of oneself and the "objective world's" perception. Horney (1950) viewed the gap between a person's "idealized image" and "real self" as a significant aspect of neurosis. Video feedback's objective quality allows a person to feel safe enough to begin to confront these differences and to begin to bridge that gap.

This is perhaps the most important quality of video feedback; it enables the client to cut through layers of denial. When confronted with a picture (worth a thousand words) of one's behavior it becomes more difficult to deny that behavior. It does remain possible, however, to deny the intent of the behavior, so there remains plenty of room to hold onto defenses if the confrontation is too threatening. This tender balance between confronting defenses and supporting the need for those defenses is much of the art of psychotherapy; the beauty of video is that it offers the therapist and client a powerful tool to sensitively explore this balance.

Video has also been discussed as effecting change through various forms of cognitive restructuring. Changes made after video self-confrontation can be attributed, for example, to an "objective shift," in which the client alters consciousness into a more objective, observing stance (Wicklund, 1975). When watching one's behavior in this state, one automatically compares oneself to an internal standard. The discrepancy between the image on the screen and the standard is often painful or distressing, and changes in behavior to conform to the internal standard may result as a way of reducing this pain. A similar, cognitive consistency theory was proposed by Boyd and Sisney (1967).

Another cognitive shift can occur when one's behavior is seen in an unaccustomed positive light. This may increase the belief that acting in desirable ways is possible in settings other than therapy; this belief may result in behavior change and increased self-esteem. Furthermore, such information may lead to changes in self-expectations and a greater understanding of how behavior impacts others. Alterations of expectations of behavior that are more in line with reality can enhance overall effectiveness, and may reduce a client's feelings of powerlessness.

Another way of understanding the effect of video self-confrontation is in relation to the repetition compulsion (for example, Spiegel, 1978). If we, as neurotics, insist on unconsciously repeating worn-out patterns of behavior in order to master them, then video gives us the opportunity to see these patterns with our defensive filters partially removed, thereby giving us the opportunity to practice new patterns with immediate feedback. From a more behavioral perspective, it is not farfetched to consider video confrontation a sort of biofeedback. We are treated to a view of our own habitual ways of responding in certain situations which in turn gives us the opportunity to modify those behaviors willfully. Those psychotherapists who view the therapeutic process primarily as a learning endeavor will see video in this light as a powerful aid to the learning process.

Other theories have been expounded to account for the apparent success of video as a therapeutic tool. Reivich and Geertsma (1968) mentioned that some clients recognize unconscious identifications with parents, spouses, or siblings during video confrontation. These recognitions can trigger insight reactions capable of serving as milestones for therapeutic change. The experience of watching oneself on the video monitor may trigger strong affect, not only in response to seeing one's own physical image, but also in response to the verbal content of the scene being watched. This affect, usually in the form of anxiety, can elicit adaptive ego functions, which in turn can enhance self-perceptions.

Another way that video effects self-perceptions is related to its tendency to magnify behaviors. This is especially true when zoom lenses are used to bring closer such things as an exaggerated smirk, angry squinting of the eyes, or nervous wringing of the hands. Zoom lenses can trespass the personal space of an individual without creating the awkwardness and discomfort that pulling a chair close to someone else might. Even without close-up shots, clients often see their behaviors magnified, helping them bring to awareness subtle forms of expression of which they may have been previously unaware.

A significant advantage of repeated video feedback is that it gives the client an increased ability to make his or her own interpretations of significant events in the therapy process, especially with the client at the controls of the recorder. Because the client feels at the helm of his or her own ship, the need for forceful confrontations from the therapist is lessened. Furthermore, repeated viewing of behavior over time gives the client a unique ability to monitor his or her own progress in therapy. Seeing improvement increases self-esteem and reinforces the progress made up to the present. The repeated viewings of particular behavior patterns also allow the client and therapist to inspect these patterns repeatedly and from a variety of perspectives. Because our patterns of behavior are multiply determined and tend to build on one another layer by layer, these various levels of causality can be examined and clarified.

Besides the implications video has for treatment, there are also implications for diagnosis and prognosis. For diagnostic purposes, video can be used to carefully compare a client's behavior under various conditions and at different times. Repeated viewing and close-ups permit careful examination of behavior which may be germane to the diagnostic process. Prognosis can be aided by an examination of how freely clients are willing to discuss their reflected self-image. Clients who are totally unresponsive to seeing themselves in the monitor tend to be poor candidates for psychotherapy; this unre-sponsiveness seems to indicate a general detachment from one's feelings and an unwillingness to confront difficulties. Both personal experience and published reports indicate that the faster clients move from the typical initial response of self-criticism to a self-acceptant attitude toward the feedback they receive, the better the likelihood of a good therapeutic outcome (Berger, 1978).

## A Brief History

The use of audiotape recording set the stage for the use of video as an adjunct to psychotherapy. Audiotape recording was seen as an innovative tool for studying the psychotherapeutic process in the early '40s; Earl Zinn is acknowledged as the first to make recordings of psychotherapy sessions. His squeaky recordings were made on wax dictaphone cylinders, which were then transcribed for the purpose of study (Gill, Newman, & Redlich, 1954). Deutsch, a pioneer in the study of verbal and nonverbal communication, used a "telediphone" to record therapy interviews for teaching purposes in 1941 (Whitehorn, 1941). Carl Rogers, however, is credited as having done the most to introduce electronic recording to the psychotherapy session (Rogers, 1942).

Moreno (Moreno & Fischel, 1942), the founder of psychodrama and sociometry, warned of the use of television as a static preserver of the culture; instead he advocated that television function therapeutically by the use of procedures to enhance spontaneity, such as those used in psychodrama. Martin, while a student at San Jose State College, introduced television to the wards of Agnews State Hospital in 1952 and began preliminary studies which were to become the foundation of the rationale to include television sets on psychiatric wards as standard equipment. He also introduced the concept of "televised therapy," in which a wide range of therapeutic programs (dance, psychodrama, individual therapy, art, and instructional programs) were presented to the patients via closed-circuit television (Martin & Over, 1956).

In 1953 Cornelison and his colleagues experimented with the use of silent movies in both teaching and on psychiatric patients; they were among the first to report the positive effects of feeding a patient's self-image back to the patient. In 1954 a French physician named Carrere published a report of his use of cinematography in the treatment of patients with delirium tremens. He made films of patients experiencing delirium tremens, and then showed the films to the patients in order to shock them into giving up their drinking.

The landmark article in the field appeared in 1960 when Cornelison and Arsenian reported in detail on their use of Polaroid photographs and movies with psychiatric patients. Photographs were taken of acute psychotic patients immediately after admission to Boston State Hospital in 1958. The photographs were then shown to the patient, and the patient was asked to discuss such topics as: Who is the person in the picture? What do you like and dislike about the picture? What would you like to change? Does the picture remind you of anyone else? Cornelison and Arsenian reported on the various kinds of responses elicited from the experience, and noted that rapid changes in psychotic states frequently occurred. Their rationale for these changes was explained in Freudian terms; because psychosis can be seen as a withdrawal of libidinal energy from external objects, photographs of the subject may be a way of redirecting libidinal energy outward because the image is of a familiar object.

Two of the early users of video feedback in therapy were Reivich and Geertsma. In a paper published in 1968, they reported on an intricately designed study of 64 hospitalized psychiatric inpatients. The vast majority reported both anxiety and positive feelings about viewing themselves on videotape, while a small portion of the patients had clearly negative responses. Despite this negativity, there were no indications of any sustained negative impact of the feedback experience.

In the late '60s and early '70s the use of video as both a therapy and training tool mushroomed. This was due in large part to the technical revolution occurring in the industry, which permitted sophisticated equipment to be manufactured at a relatively low price. It was also due in part to the works of Milton Berger, whose extensive contributions (1970, 1978) helped bring the use of video in both training and treatment to a wide audience.

In the early '70s over one hundred research and anecdotal articles appeared in various psychological journals, most of which attested to the positive effects of video. The research in this area has since been refined, although much of the research suffers from methodological flaws. Nevertheless, a large body of literature continues to grow which suggests that when video is used as an adjunct to psychotherapy, clients seem to increase desired behaviors, decrease undesired behaviors, achieve insightful conclusions about themselves, and learn new coping strategies quicker than they do with psychotherapy alone.

## The Resistant Therapist

In discussing my use of video with colleagues I have often run across the question of resistance, and it is usually couched something like this: "How do you deal with a resistant client?" or "Aren't clients resistant to the presence of video in the therapy session; isn't it an intrusion?" While these are salient questions, they may often reflect the therapist's own ambivalence about confronting him or herself in the form of video feedback. By getting in touch with one's own fears regarding the experience, a therapist can get in touch with the fears experienced by most clients, and in so doing realize the therapeutic potential of video feedback. I advise those of my colleagues who are ambivalent about using video in their work to experiment, to role play with a colleague, to watch themselves on playback, and to discuss the feelings that the experience brings up. Most therapists who were fortunate enough to have used video in their training can recall the positive impact that video may have had on their own growth, and can then relate this to the potential benefits it can have for their clients as well. Resistance in the therapist is inevitably transmitted to the client. By contrast, therapists who feel assured of themselves in this area enhance their clients' trust in the techniques the therapist chooses to use, and model comfort in taking risks, flexibility, and innovation.

## Organization

The chapters in this book are organized primarily by the type of therapy with which the activities can be used. Each chapter begins with a brief overview outlining considerations unique to the specific type of therapy under discussion, which is followed by the specific activities germane to that type of therapy. Chapters 2 and 3 respectively contain activities useful for individual psychotherapy with adults and children, while the third and fourth chapters contain activities for adult and child groups. Chapter 6 focuses on family therapy techniques, and Chapter 7 on a variety of techniques for the use of video in supervision and training. Chapter 8 discusses video use with special target populations, and Chapter 9 describes techniques requiring advanced technology. The division of the activities into these separate chapters, while usually clearcut, can be misleading in that there are many activities listed in one chapter that may be applicable in others. Where this occurs, I have tried to cross-reference. The reader is challenged to experiment, to create new activities, to pick and choose, always, of course, with the specific needs of the client kept foremost in mind.

# 2

# Individual Psychotherapy

Those new to the process of using video in psychotherapy often have questions and concerns about how to introduce their clients to this adjunct. Berger (1978) has listed four ways of introducing clients to video feedback. The first he calls *"res ipse loquitor,"* or "the thing speaks for itself." The very presence of the video equipment in an office usually spawns a curious question by the client, to which the therapist can honestly respond. The client who doesn't immediately have something to say can be queried for his or her reactions to the presence of the equipment, in an attempt to retrieve the client's fears and to work through anxiety about the use of the video equipment. The second strategy mentioned by Berger is the *"fait accompli."* The video equipment is turned on just before the client enters the session. When the client enters the room, the therapist says something like, "I thought you might like to get a more complete look at yourself today, okay?" or, "I think you're ready to risk a more open look at yourself today. It will speed up our work together." A third strategy is the "advance notice." The therapist asks the client to agree to using videotape in a following session. In doing this, the therapist stresses the therapeutic value of the technique. Although most clients readily agree, the therapist can use the client's reactions—positive or negative—as material for further exploration. A client's reaction to the introduction of video can disclose subtle issues of trust, paranoid tendencies, and grandiosity. Last is the "seduction." Over a period of time, the therapist may make suggestions regarding the use of video in the therapy session, such as, "It's too bad I don't have the video equipment here today. You really would have benefited from seeing for yourself how incongruent your happy facial expression was with the sad story you told." Another example might be to casually mention, "You know, I've used video before in therapy, and people generally get a lot out of it. Maybe in a while we can start using it ourselves." This is a technique I have often used, perhaps because it gives the client a chance to work through his or her anxieties while maintaining some sense of control.

Once video is introduced into the therapy session, it is rare that clients experience much more than slight initial apprehension. The "stage fright" reaction is extremely uncommon, and may be an indicator of severe underlying anxiety. After brief apprehension, most clients acclimate extremely well to the presence of the camera.

The therapist has primarily two roles in presenting video feedback. The first is to direct attention to cues which the therapist deems important in the playback. This can be done within the metaphor, as I prefer to do with children or with those who are particularly threatened by confrontation, by referring to the "person on the screen" or by using pronouns such as "he" or "she" when referring to the client's screen image. Pointing out cues can be done in a variety of ways. A noncommittal statement merely opening up discussion, such as "I notice you crossing and uncrossing your legs frequently," may be used. A comparison or connection between two events may imply causality and point out a client's motivations, such as "Whenever I bring up your mother you frown and clench your fists." Or, a more direct interpretation can be offered: "It seems like you get nervous whenever we talk about your mother. What about that makes you nervous?" In other words, the gamut of therapeutic interventions are available for use within the framework of video feedback, and the therapist must choose his or her interventions based on the requirements of the therapeutic relationship at the moment.

In making interpretations, a therapist should be careful not to neglect a more global set of nonverbal cues—the client's stance. This is often represented by the client's characteristic nonverbal positions: sinking into the couch as if to hide from the world, chest thrown forward and head cocked to the side as if to challenge the world, arms folded and face drawn tightly as if to put up a shield against the world.

Besides functioning as a director of attention, the therapist can be seen as providing an educative function. This consists of the therapist teaching the client to make process comments, to utilize the client's knowledge of his or her psychodynamics to self-reflect and to make cause–effect hypotheses. This is done principally through modeling of interpretations made during feedback, as well as through the simple act of observing the replay itself, that is, observing oneself naturally lends itself to making cause–effect hypotheses.

Most important, the therapist must remember that primary to the therapist–client–video interaction is the relationship between the therapist and client. Video does not dilute the intensity of the relationship (unless the therapist or client uses it for this purpose), and the client's response to the video experience will not only depend on the client's personality and defenses, but also on the quality and nature of the client's relationship to the therapist. Because of the importance of keeping the therapeutic relationship the central focus in therapy, the therapist's role may be best construed as collaborative. An attitude of collaboration on the therapist's part will prevent the therapist from losing sight of the psychodynamics of the relationship. The therapist and the client together can explore the video playback, as they would engage, perhaps, in interpreting a dream, or exploring the writing or drawings that a client might bring to the therapy session. In this mutual exploration, the therapist gently helps the client overcome resistance to examining painful or frightening beliefs, attitudes, and feelings.

Clients at particular junctures in their therapy may feel too vulnerable to withstand the impact of seeing themselves on video. The best measure for when not to use video replay is the therapist's feelings about when to use confrontative strategies in general. If, as a therapist, you would not typically wish to confront a client for fear of rupturing a needed defense, then this would determine the choice of whether or not to use video feedback. It should be noted, however, that just as it is possible to "confront with an arm around" your client, so it is possible to use video in a supportive, non-threatening manner; this can be achieved by highlighting positive, adaptive aspects of a client's behavior, and by creating a climate of confident assurance and trust within the client–therapist relationship.

The clinical research in the effects of video feedback has failed, as of the present time, to discern any specific population with which video is more effective than others. It has been my experience that a wide range of clients can benefit from the experience, from young children to octogenarians, from the mildly neurotic to the blatantly psychotic.

My work in a state hospital with severely regressed schizophrenics has led me to believe that the resiliency of this population's defenses is often underestimated; in fact, the opportunity to indulge in a bit of narcissistic gratification, such as video provides, seems to frequently outweigh fears of the unknown technique.

If a client is in an acute psychotic episode, however, video con-frontation is most likely contraindicated. It is sometimes hard to convince highly delusional clients who are terrified of being watched that the camera focused on them is for their own benefit and that the image on the screen is not being broadcast to several hostile nations. The therapist should be reasonably certain that the acute phase of the psychotic episode has subsided before introducing the video technology. I have also found that the paranoid or acutely depressed client should not be given a lot of time to mull over the idea of being videotaped before actual involvement, in order to avoid excessive anxiety or paranoid ideation. When introduced promptly and in a manner which emphasizes the likelihood that it will be a pleasant and therapeutic experience, most clients look forward to being videotaped. They should then rapidly be involved, perhaps within the next few hours, to quell any budding suspicions. The first feedback session should incorporate a host of positive (but realistic) feedback, which will result in an increased desire for further involvement.

Care should also be taken with clients who are extremely depressed, or those who have a history of depression and/or suicide attempts. It is possible that these clients may use their reflected image to validate their extremely poor self-concepts and the desire to kill themselves would increase.

This chapter contains a variety of activities suited for use with adults in individual psychotherapy. Some of the activities presented in Chapter 3 are also appropriate for adults, such as video implosion, video prep, the letter, and the monologue. Some of the other techniques in Chapter 3 may be more useful with severely regressed adults. Of interest also to the practitioner concerned with specific disorders in individual psychotherapy are the activities found in Chapter 8 on special populations, including suggestions for using video with clients who attempted suicide, or those who have seizure disorders or suffer from alcoholism or anorexia nervosa.

## The Activities

### The Naked Eye

"The naked eye" is a powerful and frequently used activity that is essentially an adaptation of the gestalt "hot seat" technique. Clients are asked to look directly into the camera lens, as if it were the eye of someone important to them. With the monitor out of sight, clients are asked to express anything they wish to the "eye" of the significant other. This significant other may be a parent, old friend, or lover, about whom the client has strong feelings that have gone unexpressed. While the direct expression of these feelings to the significant other may or may not be appropriate, the expression, and subsequent viewing of these feelings as they might be seen by another, may be of therapeutic value both as an opportunity to vent blocked affect and to discuss the effectiveness of the client's ability to express emotion.

Following this, the therapist and client review the replay together, and mutually explore the client's perceptions of how well he or she succeeded at presenting the feeling. Exploration could also deal with the client's attitudes and feelings about emotionally expressing issues to another, and how well the client's perceived expression of the feeling at the time it was recorded matched the intensity perceived by the client when watching the replay. In other words, the question of just how well the client actually expresses feeling is contrasted with how well the client thinks he or she expresses feelings. Discrepancies here may underlie many communication and relationship difficulties.

An alternate form of this technique is described by Tausig and Schaeffer (see Alger, 1973). A camera is placed directly behind a monitor, aimed at a client who is seated facing the monitor. This creates an interesting mirror, or feedback loop. The client, who is facing only the image of his or her face, is asked to imagine that the image on the screen is that of another person. The client is then asked to have a conversation with that person. The therapist, seated outside of camera range, speaks to the image on the screen, and tells the image on the screen to respond to the actual client. This creates a dialogue through the medium of the video monitor and often permits the client to express feelings he or she finds difficult to express directly to the therapist.

An interesting use of this technique has been employed by Goodyear (see Berger, 1978). She uses this technique, along with standard replay, with aged and terminally ill clients in her social work practice in New York. She finds that videotape confrontational techniques are particularly useful with terminally ill clients who are struggling with the effect their illness has on family and friends.

## The Job Interview

The job interview has been used effectively with children, adolescents and adults whose behavior ranges from the normal to the bizarre. Job interviews using video feedback are now an integral part of many job training and vocational rehabilitation programs. In these settings video is used to give feedback to interviewees on how they present themselves to potential employers and in training for maximizing their effectiveness. In rehabilitating prison inmates, for example, learning interview skills can be beneficial for the ex-con or parolee as well as for the rest of society who would rather an ex-con were employed than not.

Similarly this technique can be used in psychotherapy. If a client is changing jobs, this activity may not only improve the client's performance in the interview, but also may be an excellent way to stimulate deeper discussion of emotional conflicts. Difficulties interviewing for jobs are often representative of issues that either are or could fruitfully be discussed in psychotherapy.

The job interview is also a revealing roleplay for those clients who are not considering job changes. It can be a microcosm for many of the experiences of alienation, frustration, and impotence reported by clients. Confronting a boss, for example, may be representative of difficulties coping with anger towards a parent or parent introject. The use of this technique, both in individual and group therapy, may bring out significant issues which serve as an excellent jumping off point for psychotherapeutic work.

Speas (1979) used four instructional techniques (exposure to models, roleplaying, model exposure plus roleplaying, and model exposure, roleplaying and video feedback combined) to teach interview skills to former prison inmates. She found that of the four techniques, the video group was most successful at increasing the probability of actually being hired. The interview skills she focused on included explaining one's skills, answering problem questions, enthusiasm, appropriate appearance and mannerisms, and opening and closing the interview.

All of the inmates first completed a generalized application for employment. They then participated in a simulated job interview. The video group engaged in the following treatment procedure. A 20-minute filmed lecture was presented, followed by nine staged interviews demonstrating desirable interview behaviors. After viewing these models, the trainers divided the group into dyads for roleplaying. In the first 10 to 15 minutes, one inmate played the role of the interviewer while his partner played the applicant. They then switched roles. Following the roleplay, trainers and peers provided feedback during a 90-minute session. Following the sixth session, the videotape made prior to treatment was viewed by the group. Group members were encouraged to comment on and critique the performances of all of the group members, including their own.

Another frequently neglected group that can benefit from interview training is the mentally retarded. Elias-Burger, Sigelman, Danley, and

Burger (1981) used a standard video feedback format for teaching skills to the retarded, while Grinnell and Lieberman (1977) used a "microcounseling" approach. The microcounseling approach focused on seven specific behaviors deemed appropriate to job interviewing; these included eye contact, body posture, minimal encouragement, verbal followup, open- and closed-ended questions, and reflection of content.

A training package was used, which included verbal didactic information with cartoon pictures depicting proper execution of each skill, and modeling of the skills by a trained counselor. Each client was given two chances to attempt each skill in a videotaped trial interview. These segments lasted for approximately a minute and a half to two minutes, and were replayed for the clients afterward. During the replay, the tape was stopped each time a target-skill behavior occurred, and both social and monetary (a nickel) reinforcement was given. This reinforcement occurred each time a skill behavior was seen on the replay. The immediacy of the social and monetary reinforcement made this approach more effective than either video feedback with delayed social and monetary reinforcement, or no videotape feedback with or without social and monetary reinforcement.

Grinnell and Lieberman found that constant repetition was necessary in order for the clients to achieve mastery of the skills. Adequate time must be set aside to devote to the repetitive aspects of this program.

Another method of improving work and job-related behavior was used by Hartlage and Johnsen (1973). They used a voice-over technique (see p. 48) as a part of a rehabilitation project with hard-core unemployed clients.

**Freeze!**
The freeze technique merely implies stopping the video replay at specific intervals in order to examine the still freeze-frame image. It is ironic that the freeze-frame technique should be as popular and useful as it is, considering that in essence it is merely a confrontation with a still picture. Yet within the context of videotape recordings, the freeze-frame takes on a new meaning, because it is a still picture which can be selected carefully from a continuous flow of images that appear on the monitor. Freeze-frame permits capturing minute nuances, subtle expressions which may communicate more than a long, verbal discourse. It gives the therapist and client the opportunity to carefully explore nonverbal behavior. Watching a frozen moment gives the client a feeling of distance, permits the client to free associate to that

moment, and to explore alternate ideas and feelings which may have been unavailable at the time of the recording.

Alger (1978),* a proponent of the freeze-frame technique, considers the frozen moment to be a metaphoric experience for the client. Once a freeze-frame has been associated to and discussed, it lingers in the memory as a metaphor, an abbreviation for a variety of feelings and behaviors. Similarly, Daitzman (1977) has discussed the freeze-frame as a projective technique; by stopping an image and having clients tell stories about that image we are given a glimpse into their unconscious conflicts.

In the early stages of its use, therapists may find themselves carefully choosing the particular moment of time to be frozen. In time, clients learn to call for freeze-frames themselves. Whether the freeze is called for by the therapist or the client, the best use of the freeze is for mutual examination and exploration of the moment. The therapist should take special care to avoid using the freeze-frame as a coercive tool, that is, to show the client something the therapist feels angry about. This subtle way of incorporating countertransferential anger into the therapeutic interaction will most likely be correctly read by the sensitive client as disapproval. Mutual exploration of the freeze-frame can be an insight eliciting experience for both the therapist and the client. The freeze-frame begins as a moment for exploration, and then serves as a metaphor for the awareness gained from that exploration.

## Half and Half

Separately playing back either the sound (audio) or picture (video) portion of a videotape recording can help focus attention on attributes unnoticed when both are played back together. When listening to audio alone, one becomes much more aware of the emotion carried through the vocal channel of communication. Such things as speech nonfluencies (grammatical errors and stuttering), hesitations, changes in tonality, monotonic speech patterns, or parapraxias ("Freudian slips"), can often reveal affect hidden beneath either the content of speech or body movement. Each of these cues may be interpreted by the aware therapist, or may be left alone for the client to comment upon. The quality of one's voice itself becomes more apparent and may be a catalyst for a client realizing an identification with a significant other. (For example: "I sounded just like my mother when she used to scold

*Ian Alger has produced a 35-minute film demonstrating the use of the freeze-frame, entitled *Freeze-Frame Video*. It is available from Dr. Alger by writing to him at 500 East 77th St., New York, N.Y., 10021.

me. No wonder people are annoyed when I talk in that shrill tone of voice.")

Likewise, the elimination of the audio portion during replay heightens awareness of the multiple messages inherent in body movements. For example, a client's selective focus on the visual component allowed her to see that, although she was talking feverishly, her body was completely immobile. This led to her seeing her rigidity as a way of expressing her fear of being attacked for what she was saying. Gestures, such as a dismissing wave of a hand, or a protective crossing of the arms, may be noticed for the first time when the sound is eliminated. Repetitive movements can be interpreted in light of an attempt to work through specific conflicts, or as metaphoric expressions of particular feelings at the moment. In a group situation, the focus on the kinesic (body movement) channel of communication alone highlights interactional synchrony among group members.

Although most psychotherapists seriously consider the nonverbal aspects of communication when conducting therapy without videotape, videotaped replay with either the audio or video portion filtered out allows a more concentrated examination of the messages inherent in these channels of communication. A client's closer attention to the subtler cues used in the communication process helps the client to become more aware of messages that may have previously escaped his or her awareness.

## Videotaped Vicarious Desensitization

Combining the use of videotape with systematic desensitization procedures has become one of the most widely used applications of videotape methodology in psychotherapy. Standard systematic desensitization requires that the client imagine a series of anxiety-provoking scenes, graded according to the intensity of anxiety the imagined scene arouses. When each scene is combined with relaxation (a response incompatible with anxiety), the stimulus in the scene is counterconditioned so that the client no longer feels anxious when the feared stimulus is encountered. Wolpe (1969), the originator of this technique, lists "inadequacy of imagery" as one of the more common reasons for failure. Videotaped vicarious desensitization is a technique in which a videotaped hierarchy of anxiety-provoking situations are viewed by the client. It has the advantages over live desensitization of being consistently more readily accessible to the client, as well as being economical because the process is, to a large extent, automated.

Videotaped vicarious desensitization methods have been used

successfully to treat a wide variety of fears, including fears of taking tests (Beck, 1972; Mann, 1972), dating (for example, Curran, 1975), sexual activity (Wincze & Caird, 1976), dental procedures (Wroblewski, Jacob & Rehm, 1977; Machen & Johnson, 1974), spiders (Denney & Sullivan, 1976), and snakes (e.g., Woody & Schauble, 1969a,b).

A completely self-administered process of treating test anxiety was designed by Beck (1972). The recording begins with an explanation of the systematic desensitization method, and then gives instructions on relaxation. These instructions are also provided in typewritten form for those who wish to practice at home. The therapist on the tape then gives instructions on visualization practice, after which the anxiety-provoking hierarchy of scenes is presented. The therapist also instructs clients to turn off the set if they experience any discomfort when they visualize the scenes. There are nine situations related to preparing for a classroom examination and participating in the examination included on the tape. These scenes are presented in order from least to most anxiety-provoking and are accompanied by a five or six sentence description narrated by the therapist. These nine scenes are as follows:

1. A typical place of study with books and papers in disarray on the desk
2. A person tossing and turning in bed the night before the examination is to be given
3. The person nervously awakening and trying to get ready for class. He or she is experiencing increasing anxiety as the time for the examination nears
4. The person gathering together books and leaving for class while trying to recall everything studied the night before
5. A typical classroom with students talking nervously before class. The instructor enters carrying the examinations
6. In the same classroom the instructor picks up the pile of examinations and begins to distribute them to the students
7. Students receiving the examinations with close-up shots of an examination paper being nervously rustled by an anxious student
8. Close-up of time slipping by as the anxious student writes frantically on examination paper
9. Time running out as the last of the students finish the examination and begin leaving the classroom. The instructor is waiting impatiently for the last student to finish. Close-up of

student feverishly trying to finish and becoming more nervous as he or she tries harder (Beck, 1972).

The tapes are produced using a "subjective camera" point of view, that is, with the actors looking directly into the camera lens as if it were the client, in order to maximize feelings of participation in the scene.* This technique is effective for both individuals and groups, and can be utilized with a variety of common fears. The hierarchies can be arranged either in a standard progression as in the case above, or they can be individualized based on a specific series of fears generated by a certain client. There are some indications, however, that standardized hierarchies, specifically when dealing with test anxiety, are as effective as individualized hierarchies (Emery & Krumboltz, 1967).

Another alternative is to present a videotape of a model undergoing "live" desensitization procedures. This has been demonstrated to be effective in treating test anxiety (Mann, 1972) and snake phobias (Morris & Suckerman, 1974).

Although there is a controversy within the desensitization literature on the degree to which the therapeutic relationship is an active ingredient in the successful reduction of fears, it is my opinion that relationship variables should not be underestimated. A study conducted by Morris and Suckerman (1974) found that even within a completely automated desensitization procedure, therapist warmth was necessary to effect a successful outcome. Other factors, such as empathy and authenticity, seem to play an important role in whether or not automated desensitization procedures will be effective.

Another form of systematic desensitization conducted through videotape was described by Lautch (1970). In this fascinating case, a man who was repulsed by his own reflection was treated using a traditional form of desensitization (without videotape), after being treated by a series of unsuccessful methods. Following some improvement due to the desensitization process, the client was exposed gradually to his own image through videotape feedback. Although he resisted this at the beginning, he was gradually able to view himself when the image was greatly out of focus and in dark contrast, so in essence he only saw a shadow on the screen. Gradually over time this image was lightened and the focus improved. After 18 sessions he was able to view his face in sharp focus without any concurrent anxiety. The whole treatment, including the early desensitization techniques, took

---

*This videotape is available from Dr. George Marx, Counseling and Personnel Services, University of Maryland, College Park, Md. 20742.

four months to complete. Following this treatment, the patient made remarkable progress. Lautch acknowledges that this video feedback technique may be specifically applicable to the problems of the particular patient, but the technique may also be useful for others who have similar difficulties.

A more common fear is of snakes. Woody (1969) developed an effective, standardized videotape for use with snake phobics. The basis for the videotape was proximity, that is, each progressive one-minute scene dealt with a boa constrictor at a progressively closer distance. Woody compared three groups: one receiving traditional desensitization including viewing the videotape, another receiving no intervention, and a third receiving hypnotically induced relaxation between videotaped scenes. In both the traditional group and the group receiving hypnotic suggestions, approximately 10 to 15 minutes were spent inducing relaxation prior to viewing the videotaped hierarchy. In the suggestion group, however, clients received six suggestions between the viewing of each scene: "You can relax more; you are becoming less anxious with each trial; you take pride in your ability to relax and lower anxiety; the next time you view the clip, your anxiety will be significantly lower; your logical mind tells you that anxiety is an unnecessary response to snakes known to be harmless; when encountering the snake again you will be able to walk right up to it with no anxiety." (Woody, 1969, p. 241)

As expected, it was found that both videotape groups effectively reduced snake-phobic reactions, and that the use of hypnotic suggestions enhanced the influence of the systematic desensitization process. In fact, Woody believes that the videotaped desensitization process, unto itself, accounted for a reduction by 50 percent of the amount of time needed to effectively eliminate phobias. Woody and Schauble (1969b) also see the videotaped vicarious desensitization method as economical in that the treatment could be administered by a technician. The professional therapist would function as the programmer of the videotape and the supervisor of the paraprofessional who could present the tapes and guide the client through the process.

## Affect Simulation

Affect simulation is one of a variety of techniques that utilizes videotapes of scenes in order to prompt a therapeutic response from a client. The technique may also be combined with behavioral rehearsals of new responses, a highly useful technique in social skills and assertiveness training groups. It may also be combined with a videotaped model responding to provocative situations, in which case a "stimulus-modeling" procedure has been created (see Chap. 4, p. 71).

In individual psychotherapy, affect simulation is used to confront clients with situations that tend to elicit affect; these responses may range from a simple statement of empathy, to an outpouring of strong feeling. An actor is videotaped looking directly into the camera lens, and the client is asked to assume that the person on the screen is talking directly to the client. It has been found that most clients have no difficulty taking on this perspective. The client is also requested to experience the feelings prompted by this brief interaction, and then to introspect and explore with the therapist any new understandings or feelings elicited by the experience. The therapist who knows, for example, that a client is having difficulty coping with parental rejection, may have an older actor or actress give a hostile, rejecting message to the client. The client would then respond to this message in the safe confines of the therapist's office. Afterward, the therapist and the client would discuss the client's feelings about receiving the hostile message and the client's feelings about the response the client chose to make. If, after discussion, the client wishes to attempt a different response, the tape can be replayed and the client can practice a new response.

Another use of simulation is to pose a problem situation to the client. For example, a client may be faced with the following videotaped vignette: A physician walks up to the camera lens and says, "I have the results of the tests, and they're not good. To make a long story short, you have only two, maybe three years to live. . . . " Any number of these situations can be created to suit the needs of particular clients; the use of simulation without eliciting strong affect, however, is typically more appropriate for training purposes than for therapy purposes. See the section headed "simulation" in Chapter 7 (p. 136) for a discussion of this procedure.

## Videotaped Hypnotic Induction

Videotaped hypnotic induction techniques were originally developed to serve as a research tool, but because research on their use has demonstrated their effectiveness they are currently being used more frequently in clinical work. There is, understandably, much resistance in the therapeutic community to the use of videotaped induction procedures. This stems from the long held belief that the skill and even the presence of the hypnotherapist is the most vital aspect of successfully hypnotizing a subject: hence, the notion of "good" and "bad" hypnotherapists.

Nevertheless, research has demonstrated that even audiotape recorders can be used successfully to hypnotize subjects (Barber & Calverley, 1964); this practice has increased with the merging of hypnosis and behavioral techniques to alleviate a variety of emotional difficulties. Woody (1965) was probably one of the first to suggest that clients who have been previously hypnotized might be susceptible to a videotaped teaching induction. It wasn't until Ulett, Akpinar and Itil (1972) published a report on the use of videotape as an induction technique that the clinical application of videotaped inductions became apparent. They reasoned that an audiovisual technique presents a more lifelike and convincing procedure than a self- or technician-operated audiotape presentation. Although subjects closed their eyes early in the induction process, if they decided to peek they would still be able to see the hypnotherapist's image. Although their report failed to compare the videotape induction procedure with other methods, the authors were convinced that in their experience with over 200 videotaped inductions it represented a "good hypnotic induction technique." Further research (Bean & Duff, 1975) demonstrated less equivocally that subjects who underwent induction procedures via videotape were equally susceptible to hypnosis as those subjects who underwent live induction procedures.

The videotaped induction process generally does not differ from a live induction process except that the subject is presented with a videotape of a hypnotherapist performing the induction instead of the "real thing." Although this clearly prevents the hypnotherapist from interacting with the client, and therefore from using the client's cues as part of the induction, the procedure may have value in preparing clients for the clinical use of hypnosis, or in providing a formal hypnotic procedure to assist clients in changing specific undesired behaviors. Hypnotic suggestions dealing with weight loss, enhancing ego strength, and increasing assertiveness (cf. Hartland, 1971) adapt well to videotaped hypnotic presentations to groups.

## Therapist in Absentia

Alger (1969) experimented with keeping the videotape recorder on during a therapy session while he left the room; he then reviewed the videotape with the patient on his return. He reported that many clients behave differently when left alone with the video recorder for a few minutes, and that this behavior can be fertile material for discussion afterwards. As an example of this, Alger reported the following:

> In one session with a young man in his twenties, the therapist said that he was going to leave the room for a few minutes. When he returned, he suggested that the two of them watch a replay. The patient agreed, but immediately said, "Boy, wait until you see this." The replay showed the therapist leaving. The patient sat quietly for a few moments, and then began to grow restless. Suddenly he began to strike the arm of his chair with his fist; then, just as suddenly, as he heard the door open, he regained a benign smile and pleasantly greeted the therapist's return. It was possible to talk about the reaction of rage he had when the therapist left, but of equal importance was the new opportunity provided to discuss his way of hiding this rage from the therapist, covering it with his pleasant smile. (p. 433)

While there is no doubt that this technique may provide the therapist with excellent material, the deceptiveness inherent in the purposeful leaving of the client alone is an unappealing prospect for my own work. Therefore, I have never tried this technique. Nevertheless, in some circumstances, perhaps if it is in fact necessary to leave the session for compelling reasons, this may be a useful process to keep in mind.

The technique has also been used by some therapists in group situations, in instances where it was desirable to ascertain how a group functions without the group therapist present. In this case, the group therapy session is replayed when the therapist is present, and the effects of the leader's absence are discussed with the group members and the therapist together.

### Simultaneous Feedback

In this technique, the video monitor serves essentially as a mirror for the client. The monitor is placed so that it can be seen clearly by the client as the client is speaking. The therapy session is conducted as usual, but the client has the opportunity to see him or herself reflected in the mirror while the session is occurring. The therapist may wish to focus the client on specific behaviors of interest. For example, a client who has difficulty expressing any positive emotion may be asked to notice the absence of smiles or the presence of a fixed, pervasive, glum countenance. A client may also be asked to try to maintain a watchful eye for incongruity among facial expression, body movement, and verbal content. It is a good idea to videotape record while the simultaneous feedback is occurring, in the event that the client or therapist wishes to replay something of interest that was noticed during the course of the session.

More than one monitor may be placed at different angles to the client. Different cameras may provide the client with different perspectives. Those who have used multiple cameras (see, for example, Berger, 1978) have reported that this quite literally facilitates the ability to see oneself from a different perspective. Certain camera angles may provoke certain memories and identifications, while other angles may reflect a more customary way of viewing oneself.

The simultaneous feedback procedure helps clients get to know themselves better; it gives them the opportunity to see how they look when they express various degrees of affect in response to the therapist's questions and/or interpretations. The immediacy of the technique provides a more likely context for spontaneous insights to occur than the videotaped replay, which necessitates a certain degree of objectification and reflection.

## The Model Therapy Session

Those people who have never been exposed to psychotherapy come to an initial session with an understandable degree of trepidation. While much of this is undoubtedly due to the fear of exposing one's weaknesses and the fear of giving up or losing one's defenses, a large part of the fear in some people may be due to plain and simple naivete, a fear of the unknown.

In order to help clients who may have little knowledge about just what this strange beast called therapy is all about, some clinicians have called for the use of preparation devices. Of these, the model therapy session is one of the most desirable (cf. Krumboltz, Varenhorst, & Thoresen, 1967).

The model therapy session is a videotape recording of a "model" client in a "model therapy session"; it is shown to a prospective client prior to beginning therapy. The presentation of the model also has the advantage of providing a set of observable behaviors which the naive client may wish to emulate, thus facilitating an understanding of the implicit rules of the psychotherapeutic relationship and a shortening of the overall length of time required for a client to adjust.

## Serial Viewing

Serial viewing is a technique easily adaptable to individual, group, and family therapy. In individual therapy, the technique consists of recording whole sessions, then choosing short (five minute or so), representative segments of these sessions. The segments are either compiled (edited) onto a master videotape, or simply noted and shown in succession.

A re-cap of months of therapy can then be shown serially to an individual (or group), providing an indicator of change, as well as an overview of the process of psychotherapy. Clients who come to a point in therapy at which they wonder whether or not they have changed at all are often quite surprised to see themselves in the larger time perspective that this technique provides. This can increase motivation for further change.

An alternate strategy is to give the videotapes of the sessions to the client and allow the client to make the serial record. This gives the client the opportunity to review the process of therapy, while choosing moments in the sessions that were particularly meaningful. The reasons for the choices can be explored as the therapist and client watch the serial together. The serial also gives the therapist an opportunity to explore with the client differences between what the therapist might have suspected were significant moments and what the client chose as significant. A client, for example, may choose to focus on a particular theme to the neglect (denial) of another. This could be interpreted and explored with the client.

## Video Homework

Video homework is a way of extending the psychotherapy session beyond its confines in the office. Because videotape recorders are becoming increasingly prevalent in the home, the client may be given a copy of his or her therapy session tape to take home if compatible equipment is available. The assignment is simply to listen and watch the videotape carefully sometime prior to the next therapy session. (From the outset, videotapes may be presented as the property of the client.) Otherwise, "homework" may be done in a viewing room provided at the therapist's office. The client is asked to come to the viewing room at a prearranged time to view the tape made of the previous session (Geocaris, 1960).

Within a classical psychoanalytic framework, videotape recordings viewed at home (or at times other than the regular therapy hour) can be seen as stimuli for further free associations during subsequent sessions. Clients using the tapes this way appear to be more aware of their transference distortions, defenses, feelings, attitudes, and impulses. In general, they exhibit a significant increase in their ability to view themselves objectively.

The experience of viewing a session outside of the circumstance in which it initially occurred is not just a repetition of the original hour; it is essentially a qualitatively different session. Because the client has removed him or herself from the session by a period of at least a day, the client is able to view the session more objectively. While sitting alone watching the replay, the client's observing ego is enhanced because the client has no pressing need to defend against the anxiety inherent in the relationship between the client and therapist. This may facilitate insight.

Contrary to what might be expected, clients who are asked to expend the additional time required to come for a special homework session typically do not object. This is especially true if the homework assignments are set up as an integral part of the therapy process from the outset, much as the fee and the appointment time might be. But just as the fee and appointment time might become a source of resistance, so might the homework assignments. Anger toward the therapist might be expressed by failure to adhere to an appointment to view a videotape, or insisting that watching the tapes has become boring.

Within a family therapy context, video homework can be used to lessen an individual family member's defensiveness by giving each family member the opportunity to view the family functioning individually, without fear of being criticized by other family members. Individual viewing of group therapy sessions gives the group member a similar opportunity to examine his or her particular reactions without the immediate pressure that exists while in the midst of a group session.

## Transfer, Please

One of the advantages of using video in therapy is that it permits transfer of information from one context to another. This advantage becomes apparent when an individual is seen in both group and individual psychotherapy. A therapist may wish to videotape a group therapy session, and then bring the tape of that session into an individual group member's psychotherapy session. (This also applies to family therapy sessions.)

Issues that arise in the group may be used to exemplify conflicts currently being discussed, or manifested in, the therapist–client dyad.

A tiff that occurs in a group session between a client and another group member, spawned by the client feeling threatened by the other group member's verbal sophistication, may provide an excellent example of the anger that the client feels towards his or her parents for responding with intellectualization to the client's pleas for affection. The videotape of the group therapy session can be used in this instance to underscore the impact of this conflict on the client's relationships.

The opportunity to review particularly stressful group moments with the sole support of the therapist in such a private relationship may help a client work through difficult attempts at changing old patterns. The safety the client may feel in the individual session may give the client a chance to deal with issues too threatening to confront with other group members present.

# 3
# Individual Child Psychotherapy

To children the notion "seeing is believing" is much more applicable than it is for adults because children have a unique and sharp ability to perceptually involve themselves with the world around them. For better or worse, children spend much of their time watching television, often immersing themselves in programs to the point at which television occurrences *exist* for them in reality. Because video is so visual a tool, because the TV set is so familiar, and because it is usually regarded positively by the child, video techniques serve the child population well.

There have been no systematic studies that compare the therapeutic effects of video on children of different developmental levels, although this is a very important consideration. Both emotional and cognitive maturity will undoubtedly be reflected in the extent to which children can utilize video feedback for their own therapeutic purposes. Children who have no difficulty making discrete self–object differentiations will undoubtedly have no difficulty making sense of the object on the screen as different from themselves. Yet for those highly disturbed children who have difficulty maintaining stable ego boundaries, seeing themselves on television can be somewhat confusing.

Bahnson (1969) suggested that latency-aged children were typically too narcissistically involved to phenomenologically separate themselves from a videotaped image of themselves. Instead they see the image as an extension of a "barrierless self." In Bahnson's view, the videotape reifies infantile wishes for omnipotence, and in some cases stimulates splitting off the "bad" or damaged self from the intact observing self. The separation of this damaged self (perhaps a particularly painful introject) from the intact self, however, may be just what is called for as a part of the process of reintegrating previously conflicted aspects of a child's personality. The separation of "bad" introjects from "good" introjects is a slow and painful process because this separation can represent the loss of unconscious introjects, however despised, to which the child feels wedded for his or her own sense of security and wholeness.

At around age 8 or 9, a normal child (later ages for psychologically disturbed children) typically undergoes a process Piagetians call "decentering," in which the child becomes able to take on the perspective of another person. There is some evidence (Morse, 1976) that children who are cognitively egocentric do not benefit from video feedback to the extent that children of a higher level of development do. While children of higher levels develop better interpersonal skills after video feedback, children of lower levels do not. I have found, however, that children who were clearly of lower Piagetian levels were able to use video feedback as a way of helping themselves to separate desirable from undesirable aspects of their behavior and to increase their abilities to label their behavior, which serves in the long run as the first step toward behavior change and insight. For children who have obtained a modicum of decentering, video replay may be able to increase the child's receptivity to taking the perspective of another person. I have also found that the secondary gain inherent in the videotaping and review process has helped children to feel nurtured enough to prompt an overall lessening in resistance to the process of psychotherapy (Morse, 1978).

There are several ways of incorporating video into child therapy. One is the standard feedback technique, in which a portion of a session is played back to the child for focused discussion. Attention can be focused on recapitulating themes already discussed in the session, highlighting behaviors seen in the replay that the therapist or child may wish to discuss, or focusing on a particular behavior or theme, for example, at what points do feelings of fear emerge during the session. Another strategy is to use videotaped models in order to help the child to learn more adaptive behaviors (see p. 31). Video may also be used as a play-therapy tool per se (in which the camera is used as another, albeit rather sophisticated, toy in the playroom (see p. 39). Video games can also be used fruitfully within the psychotherapy session (see p. 51).

Video is especially useful with resistant children who see video feedback as a novelty. Children tend to be intrigued by a chance to perform on television and appear to be more relaxed than are their adult counterparts. This can be demonstrated by the ease with which nearly all children take to the introduction of video in sessions. Little more need be done than to say, "How would you like to see how you look on TV today?" and most children will jump at the chance.

Video techniques seem to have the greatest impact on children with low self-esteem, poor body image, social withdrawal, and passivity. Through repeated exposure to themselves behaving in unaccustomed and desirable ways, children begin to develop the awareness necessary to build a more positive self-concept and a repertoire of assertive responses.

I have seen no attempts to use video confrontation with autistic children or adults; without the ability to make even minimal self–object discriminations, there is no way to utilize video confrontation. There have been very effective uses of video confrontation, however, with parents of autistic and psychotic children. These sessions focus on the patterns of communication which foster alienation and withdrawal, and can have a powerful influence on the family system. These methods are discussed in Chapter 4 and 6 on group therapy with adults and family therapy.

Besides those techniques discussed here, some of the activities in Chapter 2 such as "freeze!," "the job interview," "half and half," and "videotaped hypnotic induction," may be useful with children. The sections on seizure disorders, anorexia, and Tourette's syndrome in Chapter 8 may be useful with children who have these problems.

## The Activities

### Positive Modeling Tapes

Modeling is one of the most widely accepted behavioral interventions in the treatment of many childhood disorders. Symbolic modeling uses filmed or videotaped models for children to emulate. The chief advantage of symbolic modeling is that it allows the therapist to bring situations and behaviors into the therapy session that would be impossible with a live model. For example, a videotape can bring to the session a model of a child successfully coping with a stressful classroom situation using techniques of conflict resolution completely foreign to the client. Videotaped modeling also gives a therapist the luxury of presenting a wide range of complex skills to a child. These skills can be presented systematically in a way that respectively labels, illustrates, and dissects the skill into comprehensible components. The skill can then be initiated and even practiced by the child. Essentially, videotaped modeling reduces the trial-and-error learning that characterizes most therapeutic modalities (Mayadas & Duehn, 1981).

Because videotape methodology permits erasure, the therapist can reconstruct the model scene until it is done just the way the therapist wishes it. Videotape also allows the facile use of multiple models, repeated observations of the same model, reuse of videotapes, and the viewing of models at the client's convenience (Thelen, Fry, Fehrenbach, & Frautschi, 1979).

According to Bandura's (1969) comprehensive examination of the subject, there are several factors that may increase the efficacy of a modeling procedure. The therapist who wishes to use videotaped models should keep the following considerations in mind:

1.  There should be full, accurate, discriminative attention directed at the intended modeled behaviors.
2.  Modeled behavior should be vivid, novel, and multiple.
3.  The model should have high prestige, expertise, and demographic similarity to the observer.
4.  The model should be rewarded for engaging in the depicted behavior.
5.  The model should have high interpersonal attractiveness.
6.  The observer should receive a specific instructional set.
7.  Conflicting, competing, or nonrelevant stimuli should be minimized.
8.  The observer should be given feedback and rewarded for modeling.

Meichenbaum (1971) adds a few more:

9.  Several feared objects varying in size, activity, kind, and fearsomeness should be used to increase the likelihood of generalization.
10. Modeling should be supplemented with the use of narratives. This can be accomplished either by having a narrator give a description of what the videotape depicts as well as reflection of feeling and/or instructions on how to cope with the fear, or by having the client verbalize to him or herself ("talk aloud") while attempting the feared behavior.
11. The model should demonstrate an initial fear, and an ability to overcome that fear, during the course of the modeling tape.

This "coping" model is more effective than a "mastery" model, in which the model has already mastered the task at hand.

12. Modeling should be combined with relaxation training.
13. The client should have control over the rate of presentation of the videotaped model.

These considerations are not musts; several of the above have been questioned by more recent research (e.g., Bandura & Barab, 1973; Kornhaber & Schroeder, 1975). Videotape modeling can be effective without strict adherence to each of the above considerations. A good rule of thumb is that, in general, the more similar the model is to the observer, the more likely that modeling will be effective (Kornhaber & Schroeder, 1975).

A good example of a modeling procedure was developed by DeVoe and Sherman (1978). In a successful attempt at increasing prosocial behavior in over fifty third-graders, these researchers presented the children a 10-minute videotape showing a child sharing. In the tape, the child and an adult entered a room with a second, unknown adult in it. The child was then introduced to the second adult and was told that they would be left in the room together for a few minutes. In the meantime, the child was given 10 pieces of hard candy with the understanding that it was all right to eat it while waiting. Before the first adult left, the child was told "You may keep the candy for yourself or share it." The adult still in the room with the child proceeded to talk to the child about the child's school and family experiences. The child then left the room, leaving 6 of 10 pieces of candy behind for the unknown adult. The child said before leaving, "I will share my candy with you, here are 6 pieces of candy for you." The adult said "Thank you," and the child left the room.

Prior to seeing the videotape, all the children in the study were given a sharing pretest similar in nature to the situation described on videotape, in which they had an opportunity to share candy with an unknown adult. Each child receiving the treatment then followed this procedure:

1. The child was told, "You were asked to share some candy yesterday. I would like you to watch someone else in a similar situation." The child was then shown the model tape.
2. The child was asked, "Could you tell me what happened in that videotape you just watched?" The child then discussed with the interviewer how and why the model shared. The interviewer

focused the child's attention on the fact that the model shared the candy.

3. The child watched a videotape of his or her own initial sharing situation. The child was asked to recollect his or her behavior, feelings at the time of the initial sharing, whether or not the child acted similarly to the model, and what differences were noted between the child's and the model's behavior. The child and the interviewer then discussed other possible sharing situations that might be encountered in the classroom.

4. Immediately after this session, the child was placed in a post-test situation, which was in fact a replication of the situation with an unknown adult.

This intervention procedure was effective in significantly increasing the amount of sharing in the group receiving treatment, both immediately afterward and at a one-week follow-up.

Keller and Carlson (1974) provided a simpler strategy for using modeling in promoting the development of social skills in socially isolated preschool children. These isolates were shown four videotapes, one on each of four consecutive days. Each videotape showed children involved in typical preschool activities emphasizing one of the following socially reinforcing behaviors: imitation, smiling and laughing, token giving, and affectionate physical contact. These tapes were intended to expose the children to discrete examples of behaviors which were presumed to be important components of social interaction.

The videotapes were five minutes long and were composed of several short vignettes in which a model performed one of the behaviors above in the presence of other children who responded positively. The videotapes also had a narrative sound track in which the actions of the model and his peers were described. The script focused primarily on ongoing social responses and their outcomes.

This treatment strategy was also more effective than a control, placebo treatment in increasing the number of prosocial behaviors (including both giving and receiving positive social reinforcement) among socially withdrawn preschoolers.

O'Connor (1969) found a similar procedure effective; he showed films of same-age children engaging in increasingly more active social interaction and receiving reinforcing outcomes for their proactive behavior. In each of the episodes, a child was seen watching other children interacting, then joining in, then receiving social reinforcement (for example, other kids talked to the child, smiled, and offered the child play material). The scenes varied in perceived threat from a child calmly sharing a book with another child at a table, to six children tossing play equipment around a room. A soundtrack, consisting of a woman's soothing voice, provided a running verbal description of the action in order to help the children focus on relevant cues. O'Connor found this effective in increasing the social behavior of the children who watched the models. A similar modeling procedure was used by Thomas (1974), who was able to increase attending behavior in low-income first-graders.

The uses of videotaped modeling are wide and diverse. Videotaped and filmed models have been found to be effective in reducing avoidance behavior, changing attitudes, reducing negative behavior prior to and during medical and dental treatment (see "Videoprep," p. 44), learning interpersonal skills, assertiveness, and in enhancing work and study habits. Positive modeling techniques are also highly useful in working with groups of children because they need not be individualized to each child (Thelen, Fry, Dollinger, & Paul, 1976). They are also useful for adults in a variety of therapeutic situations, and they are discussed in other sections of this book (see, for example, the section on parent training in Chapter 8, p. 160).

## Self-modeling Tapes

Exposure to television can have profound effects on children's behavior. Because of the enormous amount of time children spend in front of commercial TV, many times modeling highly unrealistic and violent behavior, these effects are often negative. Self-modeling tapes can be an effective way of using so familiar a medium in a therapeutic way.

Self-modeling tapes are self-descriptive; they are tapes of a child performing a certain desirable behavior that are shown to the same child in order to increase the likelihood that he or she will imitate his or her own behavior. The advantage of this technique over traditional modeling procedures is that because children see themselves acting in ways that are attractive to them, the identification is more intense and the goal of achieving more appropriate behaviors and ways of relating appears easier to reach. The disadvantage of this technique is that because the desired behaviors are low in frequency, the child must be able to behave in the desired ways often enough to make a useful modeling tape.

This can be accomplished in three ways. First, if the desired behavior is one which the child can role-play, the child is asked to role-play the behavior while being videotaped (Creer & Miklich, 1970). Another method is to videotape the child who may be able to accomplish the desired set of behaviors under certain conditions, and to then utilize this tape in transferring the behavior to other conditions. The best example of this is the case in which a child is videotaped while medicated, and the videotape is then used as a source of modeling when the child is not medicated and less likely to behave in an appropriate manner. The third technique is to videotape a child for a long period of time, and then edit out the undesirable behaviors while repeating the desirable behaviors. The end result is a tape which gives the appearance that the child is performing appropriately for a longer period of time than the child would be able to do naturally (Dowrick & Raeburn, 1977). When using this technique it is necessary that the end result be a silent videotape so that the behavior can be seen as continuous.

The above methods can also be combined, as in the case reported by Dowrick and Raeburn in the successful modification of behaviors in a 4-year-old hyperactive boy. An initial videotape was made of Paul's play activity while he was on medication. At this time Paul played appropriately for a short amount of time; while the videotape was made Paul was encouraged to continue to play in this manner. The tape was edited by removing nontarget behavior (the time during which Paul played disruptively) so that is looked as though Paul was playing continuously, apparently alone. Because editing out the disruptive play substantially shortened the videotape, each section of positive activity was repeated so that the duration of the task appeared realistic. A three-minute tape was therefore edited to a length of six minutes.

Paul's treatment consisted of exposing him to the edited tape prior to each play-therapy session. Dowrick compared Paul's behavior on and off the medication and after exposure to the edited and nonedited tapes at different stages of treatment. Paul's independent play behavior improved only marginally after the reintroduction to medication, and it did not increase until the introduction of the self-modeling tape, at which point Paul's self-directed play increased tremendously. With the introduction of the nonedited tape, Paul's play decreased slightly. When the treatment film was reintroduced, Paul's performance rose sharply and remained at this extremely high level even with no medication.

A novel use of self-modeling tapes combined this procedure with the use of cartoons as reinforcements (Greelis & Kazaoka, 1979). A seven-year-old girl, who was both mildly mentally retarded and schizophrenic, was videotape recorded engaging in both compliant and noncompliant (throwing a tantrum) behavior. Her treatment consisted of showing her a 30-second sequence of herself engaged in appropriate, on-task behavior. This segment was then followed by a 60-second segment of Popeye, one of her favorite cartoons. Following Popeye, she again saw the same sequence of on-task behavior followed by a repeat performance of Popeye. Following this a 30-second segment of the client engaging in a tantrum was presented. Then the client was shown 60 seconds of a blank screen as punishment. The entire sequence took six minutes and was repeated four times during each session. Treatment sessions lasted one week. A comparison of the child's behavior during and prior to the treatment confirmed both an increase in on-task behavior and a decrease in tantrums during treatment. Although this single-subject study does not imply that such a procedure may be effective in a variety of cases, the idea of splicing together self-modeling sequences with both rewarding and punishing audiovisual sequences is intriguing.

## The Monologue

The television monologue, or soliloquy, was developed by Wilmer at the Langley Porter Neuropsychiatric Institute in his work with drug-abusing and schizophrenic adolescents (1968, 1970). It is designed to help troubled adolescents articulate their feelings, to allow them to get to know themselves better free from the constraints of public interaction. The monologue is a way of both confronting oneself and of presenting oneself to a therapist.

After admission to the hospital unit, the patient is told about the monologue. Shortly thereafter the television technician on the unit asks the patient to make the monologue. (By the time the monologue is made, the patient already will have had several group-video experiences.) The technician schedules the monologue and gives the following minimal instructions: "You are to do or say whatever you wish for 15 minutes in front of the camera alone." The patient is also told that after watching the replay alone the tape will be erased if the patient so desires.

The camera is focused on the upper part of the patient's body; he or she is seated in a comfortable chair. An overhead boom microphone is used in order to allow the patient the flexibility to move about. The technician leaves the room after preparing the patient. In an adjoining room the technician starts the video recorder.

After 15 minutes, the technician returns, turning off the camera and starting the replay for the patient. The technician leaves the room again so the patient can watch the replay alone. In the event that the patient asks that the tape be erased, the technician does so without reservation.

Within a few days the patient and therapist meet, and with the patient's consent, they usually review the monologue together. If the patient wishes, he or she may show the videotape to the remainder of the therapeutic community. The monologue, with the patient's permission, may also be used for purposes of supervision and in case presentations.

The monologues took on a symbolic meaning within the therapeutic community, resembling a rite of passage from the outside culture to the ward culture. The monologue was also an initiation into the electronic environment of the ward, which incorporated television, film, and audiotape.

Patients' monologues varied immensely in topic and style, but nearly all considered it a valuable experience. Some saw it as a "confessional," using it to ease their guilt or cleanse their sins. Some patients regressed to a younger age, and others found identifications with significant others in their behavior and appearance. Most often, the monologues were bits of self-analysis, frequently with fascinating revelations and streams of associations. Wilmer noted that patients found a sanctuary in the monologue experience in which they were immune to parental surrogates prodding them on.

Monologues also can serve as records for clients who may later wish to see how they appeared when they first entered, or for subsequent therapists. Patients can be given the opportunity to make monologues whenever they feel the urge to express themselves, the way some write in a journal or create music. In a sense, the monologue legitimizes the patient's urges to express him or herself freely, and grants the patient the opportunity to act on those urges.

The treatment staff may also be invited to make monologues; typically, however, staff members are more reluctant to express themselves than are patients (Wilmer, 1970).

An alternate strategy is to have the client make 10-minute monologues instead of the 15-minute monologues discussed above. Following replay, videotape the client again, this time giving the client 5 minutes to respond to the monologue the client just saw. This 5-minute response is then replayed for the client. This alternative gives the client a chance to turn the monologue into a bit of a dialogue, and it adds a confrontative element to the process. The client is placed in the position of responding to his or her self-image on camera, thus providing an opportunity to change behavior the second time around.

## The Letter

The letter is a simple variation of the monologue. It has the advantage of being more useful for younger children who may need a more structured task in order to reveal themselves to the camera lens. A child is told to look directly at a blank television screen (the monitor) and to imagine that the screen is filled with a picture of someone to whom the child would like to write a letter. (The therapist may also direct the child to write a letter to someone else, of the therapist's choosing.) The child is requested to talk to the person on the screen as though he or she were writing a letter. The video camera is placed directly on top of the monitor so that when replayed it appears as though the child is looking directly at the viewer.

Upon replay, the therapist discusses "the letter" with the child, perhaps inquiring into the meaning of certain passages. At certain points the therapist or the child may stop the replay in order to elaborate on a particular message or further explore the motivation for a statement. The therapist also uses this time to interpret for the child and to offer supportive comments when the child anxiously treads in new water in an attempt to work through conflicts.

## Play Therapy

The videotape recorder and camera can be used therapeutically as toys in the playroom within the context of play therapy with young children. An interesting example of this use of video was provided by Heilveil (1980). A considerably nonverbal girl, diagnosed as schizophrenic, discovered the camera in the playroom. During the early stages of therapy she used the camera to get to know herself. She focused the camera on herself and watched her image on the monitor. Later, the focus on herself shifted to objects in the room. She slowly and carefully examined various objects in the room, all the while using the camera and the video monitor as her "eye." When she was satisfied that she knew the room, and therefore that it was safe, she began to use the camera to focus on the therapist. Once she was able to focus on the therapist's face and get to know it through her mechanical eye, she no longer wished to use this toy. She became more verbal, although she remained fairly regressed.

In this progression, the girl used the video to function as a bridge between herself and the world around her. The world, which was probably too frightening for her to directly engage in, was more approachable to her as a black-and-white picture of a world. Through the "window" of the video camera, she progressed symbolically through the initial stages of self-centered, primary narcissism, to the world of objects, to the world of people.

For children who may be highly unresponsive to direct interpretation, the monitor itself may be used by the therapist as a source of interpretation. A therapist can point to the monitor while the child is videotaping and make interpretive comments about what is on the screen. If, for example, a child videotapes him or herself, the therapist can look at the screen and say "The child on the screen seems to be feeling excited and happy right now. I wonder what he's thinking." This technique can be seen as "interpretation within the metaphor," in which the image on the screen becomes the metaphor for the child's experience.

Because it takes little technical acumen to operate a video camera, especially if the therapist provides it plugged in and ready to go, the camera and monitor can be used by children so inclined as a tool to explore themselves and the world around them. When conceived of as a sophisticated toy, the video camera is limited only by the parameters of each child's unique vision.

## The Mutual Storytelling Technique

The mutual storytelling technique was developed by Gardner (1971a, 1971b), as an attempt to effectively communicate with children in their own language—the language of stories and fairy tales. It is one of the techniques I use most frequently with children who have difficulty either verbalizing their conflicts directly or those who lack the spontaneity or comfort to use play to work through their conflicts. It is an excellent technique for use with resistant children.

The child is asked to tell a story to which the therapist listens attentively, all the while surmising the story's psychodynamic significance. Following the child's telling of the story, the child is asked to either title the story or to find a moral to it. The therapist then tells a story of his or her own, using the same characters, perhaps a similar plotline, and a similar context. The therapist, trying to capture the child's mood and style, tells a story that contains more adaptive resolutions to the conflicts that were symbolically expressed in the child's story. The moral of the therapist's story is the lesson that the child needs to learn in order to more effectively resolve the child's conflicts.

Although this technique can be used without the aid of video equipment, Gardner himself finds video to be an excellent way of motivating the child to tell a story. He asks the child to be a guest on a make-believe TV program. If the child accepts, as most children do, Gardner (1975) turns on the video recorder and introduces the child this way:

> Good morning, boys and girls. I'd like to welcome you once again to Dr. Gardner's Make-Up-a-Story Televison Program. As you all know, we invite children to our program to see how good they are at making up stories. Naturally, the more adventure or excitement a story has, the more interesting it is to the people who are watching at their television sets. Now, it's against the rules to tell stories about things you've read or have seen in the movies or on television, or about things that really happened to you or anyone you know.
>
> Like all stories, your story should have a beginning, a middle, and an end. After you've made up a story, you'll tell us the moral of the story. We all know that every good story has a moral.
>
> Then after you've told your story, Dr. Gardner will make up a story too. He'll try to tell one that's interesting and unusual, and then he'll tell the moral of this story.
>
> And now, without further delay, let me introduce to you a boy (girl) who is with us today for the first time. Can you tell us your name, young man? (p. 103)

Gardner then asks the child several short questions, including age, address, grade in school, name of teacher, and so on, in order to allay the child's anxiety over successfully completing the open-ended task. Gardner also plays back the responses at this point, in order to further relax the child. Gardner continues: "Now that we've heard a few things about you, we're all interested in hearing the story *you* have for us today." Some bold children will then unhesitatingly begin their story, while others are given time to think if they so desire. For children who need further prompting, Gardner adds:

> Some children, especially when it's their first time on this program, have a little trouble thinking of a story, but with some help from me they're able to do so. Most children don't realize that there are *millions* of stories in their heads they don't know about. And I know a way to help get out some of them. Would you like me to help you get out one of them?

After a positive response, Gardner continues:

> Fine. Here's how it works. I'll start the story and, when I point my finger at you, you say exactly what comes into your mind at that time. You'll then see

how easy it is to make up a story. Okay. Let's start. Once upon a time—a long, long time ago—in a distant land—far, far away—way beyond the mountains—way beyond the deserts—way beyond the oceans—there lived a— . . .

Gardner then points his finger, and nearly all children respond with at least a word. Gardner continues helping the child, by offering further prompts. If, for example, the child says "dog," Gardner responds with, "And that dog" and points to the child again. Each of the child's statements is followed similarly.

If these techniques fail to prompt the child into inventing a story, the challenge is dropped in a "completely casual and nonreproachful manner." (Gardner, 1975, p. 105.) While the child is telling his or her story, the therapist may take notes which are used to help the therapist analyze the child's story and as a guideline for the therapist's own story. The therapist also may ask the child some questions about the story and the moral, in order to clarify the underlying meaning for the therapist. Besides the story itself, the moral, title, or lesson that the child states often reveals significant underlying dynamics.

After the child tells his or her story, the therapist typically gives some positive feedback, turns off the videotape recorder, and prepares his or her own story. The therapist tells the child his or her version using the same characters but revealing a healthier adaptation. The moral of the therapist's story helps teach the child a principle that is salient in overcoming the child's conflicts.

Prior to the therapist telling his or her story, the child's story is replayed. This time period may also be used for the therapist to construct his or her story. The video replay is usually amusing for the child, and it helps the child reinforce and recall his or her own version of the story.

**Be My Guest.**   I have used several variations to Gardner's technique. In my variations I violate some of Gardner's principles, but not without positive effects. For example, Gardner stresses the importance of the child's story being a production unfettered or uninfluenced by the therapist's suggestions. I will frequently help the child who is having difficulty creating a story by giving the child a rather ambiguous situation. The video format will be a TV talk show, in which the therapist interviews the child who tells an interesting story. For example, I will set the child up by telling him or her one of the following openers:

You just came back from a safari in the jungles of Africa. You had a
fascinating experience. Tell me about it . . .

You're a detective and you're trying to solve the world's biggest
mystery . . .

You're the captain of a ship at sea. You just got back from this
fantastic adventure you had on the high seas . . .

You're a prehistoric cave dweller, and you were out hunting for food.
You came to this big cave, and you decided to explore the cave to
discover what was inside. Then . . .

Knowing the child's conflicts, I may help the child along a bit further by
inventing characters and conflict situations that the child is asked to
resolve.

Rather than leaving the child's story intact as a whole production, I
will often replay the videotape of the child's story, stopping to ask
questions and to explore alternate strategies or routes the main
characters may choose. Instead of retelling a complete story, I will often
stop the videotape of the child's story at a particular juncture, and
finish the story with a healthier resolution of the conflicts posed. If I'm
feeling very confident with my understanding of the dynamics being
expressed in the story, with the child's consent I will videotape record
my resolution over the child's. I will do this either by dubbing my voice
over the child's, or by videotaping myself telling the rest of the story.
When the story is replayed for the child, the child listens to his or her
part of the story and then hears (or sees) his or her therapist providing
a healthier resolution. This frequently provides a more intensive
identification with the therapist and seems to help the child incorporate
the therapist's resolution into the child's perspective.

Care must be taken in being sure not to erase a tape that a child feels
emotionally invested in saving. When overdubbing any of the child's
story the therapist runs the risk of the child feeling deprecated by the
therapist. This technique can be very useful for children who feel good
enough about themselves or those whose relationship with the therapist
is on firm enough footing to tolerate the high level of therapist
intrusiveness.

*Free Play.* Another variation of the storytelling technique is suggested by Gardner (1975); the child and therapist together create a
play based on the child's story. This play, which also may utilize other
members of the child's family, is videotaped and replayed to the client.
This replay can then be reviewed and discussed in order to clarify and

explore further the underlying emotional significance of the drama-
tization of the child's feelings.

*Puppet Show.* For children who are extremely camera shy when it
comes to dramatically expressing themselves, puppets can be used
equally as well. The monitor may be placed behind the puppet screen
in such a fashion that the child can actually take the audience's
perspective as he or she creates a puppet show. The replay can explore
the same issues as would be explored within the metaphor of a play or a
story, substituting instead the metaphor of the puppet show.

## Video Prep

There are many times in the helping professions when it is desirable to
prepare clients for potentially stressful, aversive experiences. This is
often the case in the medical and dental fields, where patients must
from time to time endure procedures which they might find distasteful
and sometimes frightening. Accurate information about impending
procedures helps to assuage patients' fears.

For some clients, fear of aversive procedures could be reduced by
repeated or extended exposure to the procedure without the accom-
paniment of pain. Similar to videotaped vicarious desensitization (see
Chapter 2, p. 18), clients are exposed to a videotape of the stressful
event so that when they experience that event they will be less afraid of
it.

This procedure is especially useful prior to hospitalization for
children who have greater difficulty than do adults understanding the
verbal information that is the most common form of preoperative
preparation. The major purposes of preoperatively preparing children
have been outlined by Vernon, Foley, Sipowicz, and Schulman (1965);
these include providing information to the child, encouraging emotional
expression, and establishing a trusting relationship with the hospital
staff.

Vernon (1973; Vernon & Bailey, 1974) prepared children for
anesthesia by showing them a 12-minute film of four children
undergoing anesthesia from beginning to end with little emotional
involvement. The children (both the models and the patients) ranged in
age from 4 to 9 years and were shown the film the morning of their
operations. The children intently watched the film and asked appropriate questions afterward.

Another film, prepared by Melamed and Siegel (1975), depicted a

7-year-old boy who was hospitalized for a hernia operation.* The film consists of 15 scenes showing different events that most children encounter when hospitalized from the time of admission to discharge. Orientation to the hospital ward and medical personnel, having a blood test, separation from mother, and scenes in operating and recovery rooms are included. Hospital procedures are described by the medical staff; many scenes are narrated by the child who describes his feelings at different junctures in the process. Although Ethan exhibits some anxiety in the film, he is seen able to overcome initial fears and to complete each step of the process without overdue anxiety. Similar procedures are also used to reduce uncooperative behavior of children during dental treatment (Melamed, Hawes, Heiby, & Glick, 1975).

Users of this technique unanimously report that viewing a videotape or film prior to an operation has substantially improved the pre-operative behaviors and attitudes of their young patients and has also decreased anxiety both pre- and post-operatively.

An interesting alternative which I have not seen is to prepare a child for a parent's hospitalization by showing the child a videotape of typical hospital procedures used for adults.

Although this chapter is specifically concerned with children, video preparation has also been used successfully with adults. In his research, Shipley (1974) and his co-workers (1978, 1979) utilized a "prep tape" of a person receiving an upper endoscopy examination in which a 12-mm diameter tube is inserted in a conscious person's mouth and then into the gastrointestinal tract. Air is pumped into the intestinal tract, and a physician adjusts the endoscope for 15 to 30 minutes in order to view the gastrointestinal tract. This videotape was shown to people who were about to receive their first endoscopy. In general, those subjects who viewed the tape three times experienced the least amount of distress during their endoscopy.

There was, however, a very different response between those people categorized as "repressors" and those categorized as "sensitizers" (Byrne, 1964). Sensitizers, who typically seek external information about the potential stressor as a way of preparation, showed a decrease in anxiety directly in proportion to the number of times they viewed the video prep tape. Those sensitizers who watched the prep tape three times demonstrated a smaller increase in heart rate during the endoscopy than did those sensitizers who were not prepared; those

---

*This 16-minute film, entitled "Ethan Has an Operation," may be obtained from the Health Sciences Communication Center, Case Western Reserve University, Cleveland, Ohio, 44106.

sensitizers who viewed the tape three times were also rated by the physician and nurse as less anxious during the endoscopy than those who viewed the tape once or not at all; and those sensitizers who watched the video prep tape once or three times gagged less than those who did not view the tape.

The repressors had a very different pattern. For the repressors, inserting the endoscope was accomplished more quickly in those who viewed the prep tape three times. This, however, does not necessarily relate to anxiety, for the heart rate of repressors tended to increase as a function of the number of viewings of the prep tape. Those repressors who viewed the prep tape three times were significantly more anxious during the endoscopy procedure than those who did not watch the tape at all. These findings, taken together with the results of other research, led the researchers to suggest that sensitizers "be prepared extensively and repressors left alone or at least left with their defenses" (Shipley, Butt, Horwitz, & Farbry, 1978, p. 506).

Preparation procedures are also helpful at the outset of psychotherapy, especially for naive participants (see "The Model Therapy Session," Chapter 2, p. 25). Heitler (1976) reports that preparation helps correct expectations about treatment, improves attendance, enhances progress, and reduces premature terminations. Day and Reznikoff (1980) prepared a videotape entitled "What's Therapy?" which they showed to 21 families prior to their first treatment session. The tape showed both male and female therapists in sessions with clients between 6 and 12 years of age. Parents also appeared in the session with a female parent worker. Children were shown taking part in expressive and play therapy and talking to therapists about their feelings and their difficulties. Information was also given on the videotape regarding the structure of treatment as it pertained to the particular clinic. The results of the data collected by Day and Reznikoff indicated that the video preparation group had a significantly greater number of correct expectations and cancelled or failed to show up for appointments less often than did parents and children in a control group. Notably, the videotape presentation specifically discussed failure to keep appointments as a manifestation of resistance to the therapy process. Others (for example, Long, 1968; Truax & Wargo, 1969; Stuart, 1980a, 1980b) have found various audiovisual materials, including video, film, and audiotape, effective procedures for preparing individuals, groups, and couples for psychotherapy. These tapes can be sent to a client prior to the first session, played in a waiting room, or incorporated into the first session.

## That's Me, All Right

This activity is similar to the self-modeling tapes described earlier in this chapter. The difference between the techniques lies in the fact that in this tape a record is made of a client's progress in mastering particular target behaviors. Children are videotaped performing desired behaviors in successive increments, giving those who view these tapes a sense of mastery. Tapes are replayed with pauses between each segment in order to discuss and underline children's progress.

For children who have difficulty maintaining impulse control, an initial videotape is made of the child throwing a tantrum in response to environmental stimuli. It is important to record as much of the antecedent events as possible. Incidents in which the child demonstrates improved impulse control are also edited onto the tape. This usually requires videotaping a child through specific periods in the day in which the likelihood of he or she throwing a tantrum is high. Many children have such clear tantrum precursors as being asked to complete an assignment which they feel may be more difficult than they can handle. These precursors may be used to stimulate a tantrum for the purpose of making the videotape record.

The child's videotape is then reviewed in individual therapy, with the goals of helping the child to identify those environmental stimuli that lead up to tantrumming, as well as getting the child in touch with his or her thoughts and feelings just prior to the tantrum. An effort is made to access the child's feelings of fear, hurt, anger, frustration, jealousy, and neediness, as well as some of the beliefs that underlie the tantrum. In this vein, it may be useful to discuss such irrational beliefs (cf. Ellis & Grieger, 1977) as the belief that "I must get attention from the teacher in order to know that I am lovable and worthwhile." Alternate beliefs, feelings, and behavioral responses can be taught and rehearsed with the child. These alternate responses can be edited or spliced onto the videotape over the tantrum just following the antecedent environmental stress. When the replay is seen by the child, the child sees an effective response to a potential disaster.

## Video Implosion

Implosion is an intervention that permits the client to experience the extremes of his or her fears with a supportive other present. In contrast to systematic desensitization, implosion is based on the belief that behavior change is facilitated by conditions that produce high arousal in the client. It is a way of helping the client learn that he or she can live through the feared experience without actual danger occurring, thus decreasing the anticipatory anxiety when faced with the feared stimulus in actuality. It is a behavioral intervention based on flooding; while flooding requires a client to face an actual feared situation with the support and guidance of a therapist, implosion permits the client to face his or her fears in fantasy, or at least as represented by a symbol of the fear.

Video can be used to symbolically represent that which is feared by a client. Because it is completely under the therapist's and client's control, the therapist and/or client can decide to use the confrontation to the extent deemed therapeutic at the moment. Much as a talented interviewer can manipulate the degree of stress placed on a client in order to diagnose and treat emotional difficulties in the most effective fashion, the videotaped representation of the feared stimulus can be manipulated as well.

An example of the use of video as a vehicle for an implosive intervention was provided by Morse (1978). Morse described the case of a nine-year-old child named Fred who, raped by an uncle, was unable to go to school or to tolerate a group setting. Fred saw himself as disgusting and the world as a place aimed at hurting. When Fred received any feedback that didn't match his poor self-image, he covered his ears and called himself a "shithead." His loud self-recriminations prevented receipt of positive feedback, and he lacked the ability to place himself within a time frame—that is, he did not relate to the concepts of past, present, and future.

In order to interrupt Fred's vicious cycle of self-hatred, a videotape was made of one of Fred's peers complimenting him on his swimming talents and generally calling him a good guy. When a segment of this tape was shown to Fred, he initially responded violently. Following this initial exposure, Fred was exposed to small segments of the tape only to the degree that it was not overwhelming. In time Fred was able to successfully view the complete tape. The ability to view the complete tape corresponded with a dramatic change in Fred's ability to accept others getting close to him and in his ability to seek out others' support.

The uses of video implosive techniques are unlimited; they may be applied to practically any situation that can be videotape recorded.

## Voice-over

The voice-over technique is a way of creating an interior dialogue with a child, of giving a child repeated opportunities (through repeated viewing of the videotape) to incorporate the therapist's interpretations and to learn to label affective experience. The voice-over technique was briefly mentioned in the section on positive modeling in which a narrator pointed out to the child significant aspects of what was occurring on the videotape. In essence, this technique merely calls for the therapist to record a separate soundtrack over a videotape of a therapy session. If possible, the technique could also be used with videotapes of the child in other problematic situations, for example, in a classroom or at the dinner table.

The therapist provides a running commentary on the behavior seen in the videotape. Within this commentary, the therapist calls attention to important incidents or issues which emerge and may very carefully make interpretive remarks. In doing so the therapist stays within the child's metaphor. For example, if a child is videotaped in a play-therapy session, the therapist interprets the play character's feelings and behavior. Direct interpretations are unnecessary and run the risk of alienating the child.

I have also quite often used this technique in combination with the sand-tray technique in which children are encouraged to create scenes in a small sandbox using a variety of toy characters and scenery. While the Jungian version of this technique does not call for interpreting the child's process or productions, I have found that interpreting better suits my own style of psychotherapy.

During the production of a sand-tray scene it is important not to interrupt the flow of the child's activity. Many children will spontaneously tell a story as they are creating a scene; others will work diligently but silently. Throughout the process, the child is videotaped. When the child has reached a natural conclusion, or at the end of a prescribed time, the child is stopped. I will often end by reassuring the child that his or her scene will be preserved on videotape. I may then replay the scene to the child, pausing to discuss the flow of events and the significance of the child's behavior with the child. Otherwise, I may just show the child the replay all the way through without comment.

When I use the voice-over technique, I watch the tape carefully between sessions by myself. As I do this, I narrate the child's story, interspersing interpretations of affect. This narration is recorded on a separate audio track, and the video (with the new soundtrack) is replayed for the child at a later date. An example of a narration follows:

> The monster appears from nowhere! He buries his head in the sand. I wonder what it is he doesn't want to see. Hmmm. Along comes a mountain

climber. The mountain climber looks at the monster. Here comes a tree, and a teepee. The monster's head pops up from the sand. Uh oh, along comes another monster, and he's chasing the big monster! The big monster gets bombarded by an airplane; ouch! That must have hurt. But that big monster sure can get out of hand. Hmmm. That mountain climber looks lonely all by himself. Looks like he's decided to rest in the teepee. Seems like it's real hard for him to see what's going on out there between the fighting monsters. Maybe he's scared of all those wild things going on around him . . . . Now it looks like he's gonna join the fight too, but watch out! Here comes the airplane! Whew, it missed him. Boy, there sure are a lot of things going on; it's a bit confusing. Here comes the big monster. He's trying to bite the mountain climber's head off. The mountain climber hits the monster over the head with a pick. The monster runs away. That climber sure can be brave after all! But the monster just won't quit. That monster's tough.

This brief excerpt represents the kind of narration that occurs with the voice-over technique. It seems to accomplish several things at once. First, the technique gives the child the feeling of being heard. As the therapist's words are placed on action, the story told by the child is reified, which feels validating to the child. Second, it enhances identification with the therapist, and because of the contiguity between the therapist's voice and the child's behavior, the likelihood of the child introjecting and incorporating the therapist's verbally expressed perspectives is increased. Third, it teaches the child to attach words to experience, which in the long run helps the child to communicate more effectively. Fourth, it is an opportunity to open up new channels of awareness through the process of interpreting conflicts within the child's metaphor. These things are accomplished while the child watches the replay of his or her behavior with the therapist nearby. The videotape is naturally interesting for the child and keeps the child's attention easily.

This method applies to the use of the voice-over technique in play therapy in general. A child's play therapy session can be recorded, a voice-over narration (complete with interpretations of content and affect) can be overdubbed, and the child can watch this either during the next session or between therapy sessions. Voice-over narration can be used as a way of giving positive feedback as well as a way of interpreting. For example, a child may be videotaped in the classroom during a particular activity. The therapist can then use this tape to positively reinforce effective coping skills, and to interpret and comment upon the child's motivations, feelings, and needs.

A similar technique was employed by Hartlage and Johnsen (1973) to train unemployed adults in job-related skills.

## Video Games

Video games, such as those manufactured by Atari and Mattel, can be seen as sophisticated board games. Board games, especially those with a therapeutic bent, have been used for years as standard equipment in the child and adolescent therapist's armamentarium. They are typically best used in the rapport building stages of therapy, or when a child is too anxious to cope directly with verbal interventions. In the latter case, the board game serves as a medium over which therapeutic issues can be discussed.

Electronic video games are currently sweeping the country with the same fervor that pinball machines and rock 'n' roll once did. In their home versions, they are accessible to the therapist's office. A therapist can pop in a game cartridge and use the same video monitor for the game screen as is used for video feedback.

Different video games go through periods of popularity. For a while the ubiquitous "Asteroids" was the rage, then "Pac-man" fever was something of a national obsession among children. The change in fads from one game to another may be partially due to an increase in sophistication of the games. Different games, however, attract different children. This may involve both the difficulty level of the game and the content of the game. Asteroids, for example, is a game in which children manipulate a space ship in order to blow apart floating rocks which endanger the space ship if they get too close. Undoubtedly, this game gives vent to the aggressive, expulsive impulses. Pac-man, on the other hand, is about a disembodied mouth that works its way through a maze in an attempt to eat as many dots as it can while eluding the ghosts who are chasing it through the maze. When the Pac-man eats one of the four energizers, he has the ability to chase and destroy the ghosts. It seems evident that, in contrast to Asteroids, Pac-man revels in the joys of dependent, oral incorporative impulses, while still permitting occasional bursts of aggressivity.

Video games should be used similarly to board games, although they are a bit more flexible. They can be used diagnostically, in response to such questions as how easily the child gives up when frustrated, or how easily the child copes with defeat. Does the child intentionally lose in order to protect the therapist? Does the child stare fixedly at the screen, "lost in space" (indicative perhaps of isolative tendencies)? Does the child seem too concerned with what is occurring in his or her own world to concentrate on the video game?

Video games can also be used as excellent rapport builders. The fact that the therapist is willing, and even enjoys, participating with the child in a video game gives the child a feeling of safety. Not only can the child engage in a nonthreatening activity, but the activity can be engaged in with an adult who will not banter with or criticize the child.

They can also be effective in overcoming therapeutic impasses in which the child may feel trapped between the desire to move ahead and fear of the unknown. Video games may help ease this transition by providing a safe place to make interpretations. The therapist must not be afraid to talk over the sounds of the video game; most children can split their attention between the therapist and the video game. In fact, this splitting of attention may help the child isolate enough affect (especially if the affect is being expressed through involvement in the video game) to deal, at least intellectually at first, with highly affect laden conflicts. An example of this occurred with a child who had never been able to express anger towards his parents. While playing Asteroids, and concurrently discussing an event that occurred at home, the child said, "The red rocks are my mother and the blue ones are my father." He then proceeded to intently destroy them.

Another child's anxiety was so extreme that he could not control the space ship. As an expression of his anxiety he insisted on constantly blowing the space ship (himself) up. In fact, each time he had any success at destroying the asteroids, he immediately proceeded to blow himself up. This turned into a discussion of suicide and how much he wished to hurt himself if he felt in the slightest bit successful.

Timing in the use of video games is essential. The therapist should remain aware of the fact that a child may request to play a video game as a way of avoiding the therapeutic relationship. The therapist's desire to use video may serve the same purpose, especially if the therapist feels the urge to use video instead of dealing with difficult therapeutic issues that may be occurring at the time.

A further countertransference issue stems from the fact that children are often extremely excited when they play video games in therapy. Many therapists may begin to respond more to their own feelings of rejection when the client becomes so desirous to use video that it seems to curtail open dialogue, instead of responding to either the child's great enjoyment or to the child's resistance. A child's preoccupation with the activity usually wanes after a brief period if the child is not using video to avoid the therapeutic relationship.

Another variable therapists should keep in mind is whether the child chooses to play a game alone or with the therapist. Playing alone might represent a way of working through intense anxiety for the child, but it more likely will represent a form of resistance, that is, an easy way to avoid the issues being dealt with in the therapeutic relationship. Attempts to exclude the therapist may also be direct manifestations of anger toward the therapist which should be explored in the session.

# 4

# Group Therapy with Adults

There is some difference of opinion as to the best time to introduce video to a therapy group. Most users of the technique suggest that it is preferable to introduce video at the outset of the group process (for example, Stoller, 1968c, 1970). Others (for example, Wachtel, Stein, & Baldinger, 1979) have suggested that it is better to wait until positive transferential feelings toward the therapist exist. I have found a slight advantage to working with video from the beginning, thus not having to deal with the potential complications of its entrance into the group at a later time (for example, seeing video as another group member, changing the format and structure of the group in order to accommodate the replays, and so on).

One of the major differences between using video in group and using video in individual therapy is that the process of selection of what material to videotape is geometrically more complex in groups. A primary function of any group therapist is to choose material on which to appropriately focus, and with the added use of video this becomes the function of the camera operator as well. Whether the camera person is the group therapist, an outside observer, or a group member, the task is to select psychologically relevant material. Once a videotape of a group is made, it is impossible to focus on the interaction among group members not included in the picture. This is not to say that there are or need to be specific criteria for what is relevant material. This varies from therapist to therapist and from individual to individual. In fact, as will be pointed out in the activity later in this chapter called "The Camera as Co-therapist," the choices made by the camera operator can be seen and interpreted in light of that individual's psychodynamic issues and can be very valuable fuel for the therapeutic process. In any case, the camera operator should be encouraged to avoid random photography, although random photography can never completely be eliminated.

Despite the camera operator's choice of what to focus on visually, the vocal soundtrack will remain continuous and uninterrupted. This should free the camera operator to focus on the listeners as well as the speakers. The nonverbal information found in the listener's responses give extremely valuable information for later group comment. Because movement often occurs just prior to a person speaking, the camera operator could be instructed to scan for movement in the group as an indicator of who will speak next. Movement in a listener may also be an important nonverbal comment on what is occurring in the group at the moment.

In group, as in individual sessions, playback of a complete session should be avoided, unless it is the first session. In the first session the group members may simply need to acclimate themselves to their self-images. Even during the first session, however, group members should be encouraged to stop the videotape recorder in order to discuss their reactions to a particular observation.

As with individual psychotherapy, typical playback reactions move from a more superficial examination of one's physical characteristics to a more profound awareness of one's communication style and personal psychodynamics. Over time and through repeated confrontation, clients begin to identify patterns of manipulative, self-defeating, hostile, or withdrawing behavior. These patterns can be illuminated by role-playing, modeling, and other techniques that are easily combined with video feedback. Those clients who have difficulty expressing themselves in words or who are uncomfortable in a verbal therapy mode often find video feedback a way of providing feedback about their interpersonal skills in a way that is safer and more easily understood than in talking therapy.

Stoller (1968b) discusses the necessity of training group members to "see" not only how they are behaving individually, but also to recognize the nuances of others' behavior. When a client is able to accept the fact that his or her behavior affects others and is able to understand the effect that other group members' behaviors has on him or her, the client is more likely to accept realistic feedback from both the other group members and the video replays.

The availability of other group members to reinforce the therapist's perspective or interpretations is one aspect that differentiates group work from individual psychotherapy. This group consensus function is aided tremendously by video playback. The therapist or any group member can use the playback to help confirm interpretations or offer variant interpretations. Repeated playback often serves to underscore an interpretation or to locate alternate hypotheses that are more easily acceptable by the group members. Furthermore, repeated playback confrontations are self-corrective. The group member can verify his or her behavior against three sources: self-perception, others' perceptions, and the actual image on the monitor.

Group video work seems to foster a sense of cohesiveness among group members. McNiff (1981) discussed the "ritual of playback"; over a long period of time the playback took on a reassuring, "ceremonial" quality, bringing the group together in an intimate way. The playback provided predictability and regularity. Gunn (1978), impressed with the ability of video to rapidly facilitate group process, found video to be an excellent format for providing cohesion in inpatient groups, in which the frequent turnover of group members often prevented cohesion from forming.

Waxer (1977) pointed out that group members tend to see the therapist differently after watching video replay. Video replay often affirms the belief that the therapist has no mystical power because in the replay it appears as if the therapist is doing little more than are the rest of the group members. Because of this, the therapist can use video feedback to highlight principles of democratization and individual responsibility in group functioning. This, however, can lead to the danger of deluding oneself as well as the rest of the group into thinking that video feedback is free of transferential qualities. In fact, no matter how democratically the therapist wishes to introduce the use of video feedback, it is most often under the therapist's control. Even when other members of the group are encouraged to use the equipment freely, it is the therapist who knows and understands the equipment best, and, perhaps after substantial experience, feels most comfortable with its use. Consciously or unconsciously, many group members will see the videotape methodology as powerful extensions of the therapist's authority. Lack of awareness of this on the therapist's part may paradoxically lead to an increase in the transference and a concomitant increase in the therapist's difficulty in understanding and utilizing that transference (Wachtel, Stein, & Baldinger, 1979).

Resistance to being videotaped or to watching a playback should be understood in the same manner as is resistance in any form. Generally, the rights and dignity of every client to avoid self-confrontation should be respected and should be seen as clear messages of vulnerability and need for distance. If the therapist is concerned that interpreting or pushing the resistance would be countertherapeutic, the therapist may decide to allow some members to sit out of the range of the video camera if they do not wish to be recorded. This will usually desensitize resistant clients, while permitting the client to interact with the other group members who will probably be interpreting and working with the outcast client. Those who offer strong resistance may be indicating a defensiveness strong enough to preclude them from being involved in the group; these group members would probably eliminate themselves from group regardless of the presence or absence of the video equipment.

An obvious consideration, but one that is important to note, is that group members will follow the style and the tone of the group leader in deciding how to interpret the playbacks. The group leader should therefore set a tone of support combined with realistic confrontation; this will do much to prevent destructive criticism by the group members (Katz, 1975).

There are several factors which can help to achieve acceptance of video as part of the group therapy process. Perhaps the most important of these is the degree of acceptance and comfort the therapist feels with the use of video, the level of which will undoubtedly be communicated to the group. In addition, making the parameters of video use extremely clear at the outset of therapy tends to decrease resistance. The therapist should come to an agreement with the group on issues of when the group will be videotaped, and most important, who if anyone else will see the videotapes. Consent must be obtained for showing the videotape to others, and if there is any doubt about exactly how the tapes will be used, formal releases should be signed by all group members.

Other considerations include placing the camera where it is visible to group members. If the therapist wishes to have an outside observer or technician doing the videotaping, this must be presented to and agreed upon by the group. It helps to present the camera person in a legitimized role (Hadden, 1956), similar to presenting a supervisor, guest therapist, or student. In fact, Mayadas and O'Brien (1973) have reported much success at combining the two roles of student observer and camera operator.

In this chapter the reader will find activities applicable to use of video within the context of a private practice and within the context of a hospital unit. Video as it is combined with movement and art therapies as well as with psychodrama is also discussed. Some of the activities in this chapter are adapted for use with video from gestalt techniques and human relations training; the group leader familiar with these techniques may find many others that are suitable for use with video.

Some of the techniques listed in Chapter 5 on group therapy with children may be applicable to some adult groups, especially those which have low-functioning members. Furthermore, many techniques in Chapter 2 are also adaptable for use in groups. The section on assertion training in Chapter 8 may be particularly useful for group therapy facilitators.

## The Activities

### The Hospital TV Station

Despite significant budget cuts in California's state hospital system, Camarillo State Hospital in southern California has been operating an in-house television station now for more than 15 years. This innovation began operating under the auspices of the Rehabilitation Service of the hospital for the purposes of creating and broadcasting its own programs. When the station began operating in 1962, it was staffed by 40 regressed patients. Two staff members currently supervise the station which is operated almost exclusively by hospital patients. The unique aspect of this station is that it broadcasts on a separate channel to all the wards in the hospital. For quite some time it has broadcast both educational and entertainment programs of its own devising. These programs include a daily newscast in which hospital activities for patients are advertised, exercise programs, variety programs featuring patient talent, discussions, interviews, concerts, religious programs, and telecasts of local sports events. Hospital patients may choose to watch this station or to watch any of the commercial stations available to them (Emmitt, 1981).

But the purpose of the station is twofold; besides operating as a highly successful industrial-therapy program for patients, it is also a part of the hospital's therapeutic program. Currently, Dr. Ira Greenberg conducts a psychodrama session in the studio which is taped for broadcast to the hospital wards just two hours later. This form of open therapy was originated at the hospital many years earlier by Dr. Vogeler who conducted regularly scheduled psychodrama sessions for broadcast to the wards.

Dr. Frederick Stoller (1978a) continued this initial experiment, leading group volunteers chosen from among the hospital's most severe, chronic population—patients judged by the staff as making no progress despite years of hospitalization. The original ten female patients sat in a close circle with two video cameras that could move around the periphery. In this initial group, Stoller focused on enhancing interaction among group members and toward others in their environment, the patient's static, "institutionalized" stance, and patients' poor self-concepts. A strong emphasis was placed on changing current passive attitudes. Stoller witnessed a marked improvement in the behavior of these chronic patients, some of whom had been in the hospital for as many as 14 years. Over time delusional verbalizations decreased. The most striking change that Stoller reports was the improvement in the level of the group's spontaneity. Some of the patients were motivated to seek off-ward industrial therapy, and many began to seek out hospital activities they heretofore had ignored. Some improved enough to leave the hospital.

It is impossible, of course, to determine why these changes occurred. Other patients, particularly those from the group members' home ward, responded to the group members with excitement and recognition. Staff also began to treat these patients differently. Both staff and patients commented positively about the group members' behavior and their physical appearance. Staff members treated the group members differently due to their surprise at how well they performed. The video feedback appeared to enhance the natural group tendency toward guiding the members away from pathology. Being a participant in a group broadcast to the hospital wards gave patients the opportunity to cooperate with others in performing before the world at large.

These changes seemed to last even when the novelty of the experience wore off. In time, as patients left the group and new patients were added, the format of the group began to change. Other groups were added. One of the changes was the opportunity for the group members to view their own videotapes and to discuss their impressions immediately afterward.

There was a further advantage to the broadcast of the group therapy sessions to the hospital units; it apparently helped the audience as well as the participants. The close-up shots seemed to foster intense identification. Seeing others with such similar issues work these issues through provided a vicarious therapeutic experience.

Stoller also makes a strong point about the positive impact the televised groups had on him as a therapist, and on the positive impact he suspects it would have on the profession as a whole. The ability to see a psychotherapy session conducted demystifies it and relieves the potential client of fears of being overwhelmed or devastated by the process. Stoller feels that many psychotherapists unwittingly perpetuate the conception of psychotherapy as an arcane art in order to perpetuate their own needs for omnipotence. He noted that it was much easier to get patients to participate in this activity than to get other therapists involved.

## Psychodrama and Video

*General Considerations.*   Psychodrama and video feedback are natural bedfellows. Hollander and Moore (1972) point out that both psychodrama and video self-confrontation have similar origins and goals. In fact, the founder of psychodrama, Jacob Moreno, was also one of the first to incorporate video into his form of group therapy. Both video feedback and psychodrama use the tools of the entertainment and communication media to accomplish their goals, though both use these tools in a way very different from the commercial theater and communication industry. While the entertainment media provide imitations of life in order to remove the audience briefly from their real lives, both video feedback and psychodrama encourage the audience to heighten awareness of the here and now. In psychodrama, history and future both come alive in the present. In video feedback, the past happens in the here and now. Each time the tape is replayed past actions recur and the scenario of the past is reenacted in the present.

Both psychodrama and video feedback attempt to achieve spontaneity in participants. In psychodrama, the participants are asked to flow with the action that emerges moment by moment, while the audience is asked to freely react to the enactment, share in the production, and share its reactions. In video feedback, the spontaneous behavior of those before the camera is the most fruitful source of feedback.

Hollander and Moore see democracy as the essence of both psychodrama and self-confrontation via video. In psychodrama the attempt is made to focus on a topic and protagonist that is the democratic choice of both the audience and the volunteer protagonist. They see video feedback as promoting more democracy than any other form of therapeutic adjunct, primarily because the client has access to the same information as does the therapist. The client becomes co-diagnostician and co-therapist when watching video feedback. Furthermore, if the therapist's behavior is also videotaped, the therapist's behavior is as available for consideration as is the patient's.

Video feedback allows the psychodramatic protagonist to become his or her own audience, an element which psychodrama without video lacks. Because the protagonist is on stage, he or she does not have the choice to simultaneously act and be in the audience. This limits the therapeutic learning to catharsis and the protagonist's ability to assimilate information from the director and auxiliary egos. Because of the heightened emotional involvement of psychodrama, the protagonist's ability to consider all the data that emerged from the integration phase of the psychodrama is limited. Viewing the videotape of the psychodrama afterward permits the protagonist to become part of the audience and to augment his or her integration of the enactment.

Hollander and Moore recommend that a smoothly functioning psychodrama enactment not be interrupted for video feedback. Video feedback can serve an important function by stepping in at the point at which a psychodrama may be breaking down, either because of resistance from a protagonist or because of inept direction. The director may interrupt the psychodrama and, with the group, may try to ascertain the reason for the failure of the session to move properly. Replay of the warm-up tape possibly can help to uncover inadequacies in the warm-up phase such as dissatisfaction with the choice of protagonists or the director's predetermined choice of direction.

Video can also serve as feedback for the director. Because the psychodrama director is often alone, he or she has few sources of adequate feedback or supervision from colleagues who may not be trained in psychodramatic techniques. Video feedback permits the psychodrama director to remove him or herself from the midst of the action in order to view his or her directing technique at a later time when it is easier to be objective (Goldfield & Levy, 1968).

**Warm-up.** A technique for warming up psychodrama participants to their personal concerns is to have the group member sit facing the video monitor while the monitor simultaneously feeds back the video portion without sound. The participant is encouraged to conduct a verbal monologue, asking questions such as, "What do you think of the person on the screen?" or "What does the person on the screen feel right now?"

**Mirroring.** In psychodrama, mirroring refers to a protagonist being pulled from the action in order to watch an auxiliary ego go through the protagonist's motions. This perspective may also be accomplished by the protagonist's reviewing the video replay of the preceding few minutes of the psychodrama.

***Delayed Feedback.***   More standard forms of video feedback can be used after the psychodrama has been completed. Because the protagonist may need several hours (or, in some cases, several days) to wind down, the feedback session can be conducted with the protagonist after such a delay. Here the intent is to help the protagonist to further integrate new awareness about his or her previous performance. The protagonist should be asked what portions of the psychodrama he or she would like to see replayed, a process which gives the therapist important clues as to which meaningful conflicts were left unresolved. During this replay, a protagonist may be given a second chance at assimilating input from other members of the psychodrama, or contradictory or incongruent verbal and nonverbal messages may be pointed out. It is suggested that the therapist only focus on a few specific instances during the replay in order to avoid emotionally overloading the client. Following this, the client may wish to view the complete psychodrama once without stopping in order to increase a sense of closure.

***Audience Replay.***   Audience participation in psychodrama is usually elicited through the final, sharing stages. Often, it is difficult for audience members to remember how they felt about a specific instance. Just as it can be used for replay to those in the group as a whole, or to individual members of the group (including the director), video feedback can be of value to the audience. This requires that audience reactions be videotaped during a psychodrama. By reviewing their reactions, the audience is placed "on stage," and the audience can see themselves as actors as well.

## The Camera as Co-therapist

In this activity, a particular group member operates the camera for the duration of a complete therapy session. Over a series of group therapy sessions, group members alternate acting as camera operator, each having his or her turn. The goal of this activity is not only to provide a source of group feedback for the group as a whole but also to provide feedback of the group as it is specifically seen by the camera operator, that is, by a particular member of the group.

A brief orientation to the operation and function of the video equipment is necessary and should probably be done with the group member prior to the beginning of the session. This reduces the client's anxieties and makes for smoother taping of the sessions.

The method used for selecting the camera operators may vary; whether the group member volunteers on a specific day, is assigned ahead of time, or rotates through seems to have little impact on group function. Each method will have its implications for group process, however, and may provide substantive issues not to be ignored.

Both the general content and the perspective of the camera operator are examined as part of the feedback process. Initially, the therapist serves as a model for interpreting the choices of the camera operator, but soon afterward the group members become involved in interpreting the camera operator's choices as well. While that which is recorded serves as an important base for interpretation, that which is not recorded is also noteworthy. Positive and negative transferences, unresolved conflicts, affectional and hostile relationships emerge in the camera operator's choices of whom to focus on and the length of time on which each group member is focused. Another choice that has a clear symbolic implication could include the camera operator abdicating his or her role by placing the camera far away from the group and videotaping the whole group at once. Clearly, this may indicate not only a desire to join the group but also a desire to hide from the threat of being available for interpretations. Focusing on a particular group member for an inordinate amount of time may reveal an interest previously unexposed, and the pattern of movement from one group member to another may reveal a particular pattern of transferences, such as one's family constellation.

Heckel (1975) has found this technique useful for all age groups, including adolescents and children. He originally described the technique, and it has been developed using the suggestions of Mervyn Wingard.


## Doubling Playback

Those who are familiar with the techniques of psychodrama will be familiar with doubling. The activity that follows is an adaptation of the doubling technique—described by Richard Lee of the Family Institute of Cambridge (Lee, 1981)—and is for use with video feedback that can easily to be incorporated into most group therapy formats.

The therapist replays a portion of a videotaped interaction and instructs the group members to call for a stop in the tape simply by beginning with the words "As myself . . . " and then saying what he or she may be feeling but not saying on the tape. While a group member may wish to do this in order to amplify or clarify a feeling he or she may have at the moment, a particular group member may wish to "double" for another group member, by saying, "As Mary (the other group member), I . . . " The person who is spoken for may wish to use what is said by the other group member about him or her or to change it and put it into his or her own words. After a comment is made by a double, the person being doubled for is given a chance to speak if he or she so desires.

The therapist who is conducting this exercise should do it slowly, modeling the process of doubling if the group members are slow to respond. The therapist may wish to model by making comments such as, "As myself, I'm wondering why I didn't ask John how he was feeling. I guess I was afraid John may have been wanting time to himself and I didn't want to interrupt that," or, "As Mary, I'm feeling angry at myself that I didn't tell John how I felt when he said that about his girlfriend."

## Blindfolded Block-stacking

Blindfolded block-stacking is a good warm-up activity for use in the early stages of group therapy. It focuses on such issues as helping versus helplessness and dependence versus autonomy. It requires the following materials: a box or bag of children's wooden blocks, blindfolds for the group participants, and a clock or watch with a second hand. The blocks are poured into a pile in the center of the floor. Two group members are asked to sit facing each other with the blocks between them. The camera is placed so that the profiles of the group members are videotaped. The participants are told that the game should take approximately ten minutes and that the objective is to build a stack of blocks as high as possible and to leave it standing at the end of two minutes. The group facilitator will then count how many blocks are on top of each other in a column. Several blocks may be placed horizontally in order to support the structure, but only the height of the structure will be measured. The group may wish to see a demonstration at this point, and the therapist may wish to demonstrate by building a tower and counting the number of blocks in a single column. After making sure that the instructions are understood, the group leader tells the group that in order to make the activity more interesting, the participants will be blindfolded, and the videotape recorder will allow the participants to watch the event afterward.

The volunteers are then blindfolded, and they are asked to place their strongest hand behind them. After adjusting the blindfolds, checking the watch, camera, and recorder, the players are told to begin. The two participants will undoubtedly construct two towers on either side of the pile. At the end of the two minutes the participants are told to stop and to remove their blindfolds. The number of blocks in each tower is then counted.

At this point the therapist may wish to discuss the preceding event or go on to the next two players, postponing the discussion and feedback until the end of all three rounds.

The group members are then asked to do this activity again, a bit differently. This time only one member of the group builds the tower while another group member, not blindfolded, serves as the helper. The helper may not touch the stack of blocks but must only help by conversing with the stacker.

The therapist asks which person would like to do the stacking and which person would like to do the helping. This time the camera should be focused on the tower and face of the helper. After two minutes, the stacker removes his or her blindfold, and the blocks are counted. Now the stacker and the helper are asked to switch roles. These two minutes are also videotaped, focusing on the tower and the helper's face. Following this last round the participants are asked to discuss what it felt like to build the tower. They are asked to discuss which of the rounds was most enjoyable and which was least enjoyable and how it felt to help and be helped. Further discussion centers on what experience, if any, the participants were reminded of in their lives. The videotape is rewound to the beginning of the first round, and the other group members are asked to comment on the behavior of the players. Such issues as willingness to ask for support, dependency, intimacy, fear of failure, and competition emerge from this activity.

Variations of this activity permit more than two players. In the second and third rounds, each player chooses a partner and a role. More than one helper is permitted. Several triads may be formed within a large group, with two players and a director in each triad, possibly switching roles. At the end of several rounds, the videotape (or tapes) should be rewound and replayed, with the complete group available to make comments.

This activity was first devised by Rosen and D'Andrade (1959) in order to experimentally demonstrate motivation for achievement in children. It was adapted by Lee (1981) for use in group and family therapy.

## Speed Shift

Most video recorders have the capability of shifting the speed of the video playback. Slowing or speeding up the replay can highlight patterns of interaction that may go unnoticed when seen at standard speed. By speeding up the replay, some patterns of nonverbal behavior may become clear that cannot be seen at standard speed. For example, one couple noticed the tremendous discrepancy between husband and wife in the amount of nonverbal movement when the tape was played back at faster than normal speed. The great movement of the wife was exaggerated against the almost complete stillness of the husband which led the wife to recognize her chronic anger at her husband for his general unresponsiveness to her needs (Alger, 1969).

At slow speeds, rapid movements which may go generally unnoticed become more available for scrutiny. A quick downward glance on slow motion may reveal shame which was not apparent or conscious when it occurred initially. A brief gesture, which may have seemed to have little or no significance when it occurred, upon slow motion replay may reveal an obscure meaning. A group member who quickly wipes his nose with his finger while another person is speaking may see that gesture in slow motion as a message of disgust.

Both slow and fast motion replays may also reveal a certain "interactional synchrony" among group members, a series of rhythmic, coordinated movements indicating empathy between two or more members. This synchrony may not be apparent during the replay at regular speed because attention may be focused on other aspects of the replay at the time. The distortion inherent in changing speeds permits relationships among group members to "jump off the screen" to a greater degree than when watching a replay at normal speed.

## Sorry I'm Late

Many latecomers to a group therapy session, especially those with paranoid tendencies, fear that the group has used the group member's brief absence as an opportunity to talk behind his or her back.

A group member who comes to a videotaped group meeting late is asked to talk about his or her fantasy of what occurred prior to the group member's entrance. The latecomer who verbalizes beliefs that his or her absence was either completely ignored or used as a chance to criticize, can be helped by replaying the videotape of the session that occurred prior to the group member's entrance. During this playback, the group's expressions of caring concern cannot be easily refuted by the client, who may be surprised to see that the others care enough to worry. This experience, in turn, may help the group member to feel more at ease and to trust others and express affection.

One difficulty with this intervention is that it requires that the group members have in fact responded positively to the group member's absence. If hostility was expressed, the therapist may, of course, choose to either not ask the client for his or her fantasy or replay the earlier section of videotape, unless this confrontation with the group's anger is deemed by the therapist to be appropriate or helpful. This depends on the therapist's interpretation or understanding of the group member's motivation for his or her lateness.

Replaying the early portion of a group to someone who was not involved in the group process at the time gives the rest of the group the opportunity to receive feedback from a person who, because of his or her lack of involvement at the time, may be able to respond more objectively. This activity was developed by Berger (1978).

## As the World Turns

Lazarus and Bienlein (1967) devised a simple technique which uses brief portions of soap operas to stimulate group process. Soap operas can be extremely useful when dealing with resistant clients or with clients who for any reason may be too threatened by the prospect of group therapy to confront it directly. Those clients, particularly institutionalized ones who have "had it to here" with psychotherapy, often respond well to the vicarious thrills afforded them through the viewing of soap operas.

The first 15 minutes of each group session is devoted to watching a single episode of a soap opera. After watching the episode, each group member is asked by the group leader to choose a particular character or situation for discussion. The group leader attempts to accomplish three things at this point: to help clients articulate what has actually been perceived; to have clients relate their perceptions of the soap opera to personal experience (thereby helping clients to understand the rationale for perceiving the situation in their unique way); and to stress the importance of expressing one's feelings in interpersonal relationships. The leader functions, at this point, more as a teacher in expressing one's feelings, and in so doing uses concrete examples from the lives of the group members as stimulated by the soap opera. Lazarus and Bienlein require each group member to participate in turn.

Following this discussion, the second portion of the group is devoted to more traditional group therapy, using the prior discussion as a foundation. This section remains more flexible and dependent on the group's needs.

Lazarus and Bienlein found that watching the soap opera markedly freed the group members to discuss themselves in ways they were extremely reluctant to do beforehand. "It was as though merely viewing the problem in this projected form sufficed to legitimize it as a subject for discussion" (p. 254). There are several other reasons that soap operas are valuable in group therapy: They allow the client to be involved in an affect-laden situation without having to participate directly; they decrease the frustration therapists may experience with passive and resistant clients, simply because clients tend to be less passive when involved in this activity; they allow the therapist who knows the dynamics of particular clients to make metaphorical interpretations (that is, to point out conflicts occurring within the soap opera that may be relevant to particular clients without necessarily labeling them as that client's conflicts); discussion of the soap opera can be used to protect a scapegoat or limit a monopolizer (by shifting the focus toward or away from the client and onto the next client); and, despite the fact that many of the models are less than desirable, it is a useful didactic device for teaching principles of emotional conflict, motivation, assertiveness, communication, and catharsis.

A therapist may use the attention, or lack of it, that a client pays to the soap opera as an indicator of the client's emotional state. For example, if a client becomes preoccupied at a particular moment while viewing a soap opera, the therapist might ask the client what the last thing he or she remembered before becoming preoccupied. This gives the therapist and client a valuable clue as to the particular conflict the soap opera elicited for the client at the time.

Soap opera segments should not be overused. After several sessions group members often feel that they no longer need the stimulus of the soap opera and may prefer more conventional group therapy.


## Video Art Therapy

Since its inception, video has been a tool for artists as well as for psychotherapists and commercial television producers. Video art has been exhibited internationally, and a recent search of the holdings of the University of California listed over 40 books on the subject. Video has also been used as an art therapist's tool, extending the resources of the art therapist beyond the traditional devices of drawing, painting and sculpting.

There are many ways in which video can be incorporated into art therapy. One way is to encourage clients to use video to create their own productions, thereby capitalizing on its potential for creating a sense of self-worth and fostering spontaneous expression and catharsis. Discussing the product and the process with the client also yields insight. For example, a production that is fragmented and unfocused in its content may represent a client's feelings of confusion and anxiety, while a production that is smoothly and crisply edited may represent coherent and unconflicted thinking.

The chief difference between most forms of video feedback and video art therapy is that in video art therapy the record made by the camera operator is primarily subjective (McNiff and Cook, 1975). The camera operator is encouraged to edit in-camera, and to record his or her personal perception of the event being recorded.

As with any form of art, video is a projection of the artist's personality. It is easy to forget this when watching videotape due to the feeling of objectivity inherent in watching something that has become fixed onto the videotape. One should keep in mind the idiosyncracies that define an individual artist's conception of the world; an over-abundance of close-ups or long shots may represent the individual's struggles with intimacy, as may a quick, fleeting transfer from one shot to another. A group member focusing purely on interactions may represent intrigue with interpersonal issues, while a focus on facial expression may represent an overconcern with affect. The unique ways in which an event is seen by an individual are rich fuel for discussion in a group format.

The video art groups conducted by McNiff and Cook at Danvers State Hospital begin with informal socialization while the video equipment is set up. Group or individual art activities are then conducted and taped for later playback. After approximately 45 minutes the group takes a break and returns to view the playback. Due to the fact that the camera operator has only selectively recorded the art therapy activities, the final videotape is only between 10 and 15 minutes long. The brevity of the tape also prevents overstimulation. The tape is played, stopped, and replayed as discussion warrants. Finally, a discussion of the complete experience is held. This too is videotaped and is frequently played back. The complete session lasts between two and three hours.

Of the many activities used in their groups, McNiff and Cook often provide a basic structure through the use of creative movement exercises. They present such simple themes to the group as walking, slow-motion touching, jumping, interaction, and power at the beginning of the session. Individual and group activities are then developed spontaneously as they relate to the chosen theme. They also use such props as rope, foam rubber, and string as a way to build a communal environment. Auditory perception is developed by experimenting with voices and objects found in the environment. Their groups have also videotaped community activities, including people's responses to art exhibits.

Because their groups have a strong emphasis on perceptual development, group members are encouraged to discover visual and auditory relationships as they are presented in the playback. Visual memory can be tapped by asking such questions as, "Can you duplicate the gesture made by Tony when we were doing mime?" while auditory memory can be tapped by asking questions relating to recalling what was said at a specific moment during the group. More affectively toned auditory or visual memory can be developed by centering the discussion on such questions as, "Did the playback accurately represent your feelings at the time?"

## The Individual Portrait

The individual portrait can be a very valuable exercise within a group therapy context, especially for clients who have highly distorted self-concepts or those who have great difficulty expressing themselves to others in the group. This activity is particularly useful in groups conducted in hospital settings where more severely disturbed and nonverbal clients are more likely to be found.

The individual portrait usually involves either a client or a therapist videotaping a client engaging in a specific activity. This may be an interaction between client and therapist or it may be an interaction chosen by the camera operator for its symbolic value. The videotape is then shown to the entire group. The group members are encouraged to discuss the portrait, and to offer their insights and interpretations concerning what they see in the client. The reasons that the camera operator chose to focus on particular aspects (for example, a close-up of a facial expression) and not others could also be explored in such a context.

Variations in this technique include an individual group member making a self-portrait outside of the group which the group member brings to the group for discussion. Another variation is to have two group members working together on one portrait. Each partner is encouraged to make a portrait of the other as he or she is seen by that group member. These portraits are then shown to the remaining group members who offer their own perceptions and clarifications.

## Stimulus-modeling Tapes

Stimulus tapes can be used to elicit group reactions, or they can be used more specifically with the goal of modeling new behaviors. In the latter case, a particularly provocative situation may be presented on videotape along with a model who copes adaptively with that situation. Stimulus-modeling procedures are best used in small groups focused on a specific topic. For example, they are extremely useful in parent training, assertion training for adults and children, educational or consciousness-raising groups for women (and men), groups formed to discuss issues of death, dying, or loss, social skills training, and in the training of clinicians.

Mayadas and Duehn (1981) have outlined some specific considerations relative to the use of stimulus-modeling procedures. It is important that the video presentation be clearly focused on the immediate areas of concern, whether they be affective or behavioral in nature. The stimuli presented in the tapes should lucidly identify specific contextual antecedents which may (or may not) give rise to the problematic behaviors. If the behavior to be modeled is complex, it should be presented in a fashion that permits sequential approximations of the behavior. This prevents the client from becoming overwhelmed with the complexity of the task and thus tuning out.

Once you are aware of the behaviors on which you wish to focus, there are essentially three ways to present these behaviors for videotaping: use of a studio to enact the behaviors; use of the natural environment; and use of the clients themselves in either a studio or natural environment. Each method carries with it advantages and disadvantages. Recording in a studio allows for greater control of the production. After writing a script or outline, actors are coached to enact the situation to the therapist's standards. Studio work permits a greater degree of comfort and customization of the product. Both actors and situations can be tailored to be as similar to your client groups as you wish. There are also fewer distractions that may impinge on the isolation of the task to be learned. Also, tapes made in a studio may be high enough in quality to be made available to colleagues and educators who, as part of a library or commercially, may wish to use the tapes for similar purposes. The disadvantages of working in the studio include limited access, high production costs, and time restriction.

Producing tapes outside of the studio, in the natural environment, gives the final product greater authenticity. This enhancement of authenticity may come at the expense of lower quality tapes, however— a result of the typical lower quality equipment used for on-location shooting at the amateur level. Furthermore, it is difficult to control the intervening and potentially distracting stimuli that may impede the isolation of the target behaviors.

Use of clients to model themselves is another option. This is less appropriate in a group therapy context than it is in individual therapy, and is discussed in the section entitled "Self-modeling Tapes" in Chapter 3, p. 35.

Mayadas and Duehn discuss a "standard format" for combining stimulus-modeling tapes with other such commonly used techniques as behavior rehearsal, video feedback, and homework. This format includes the following steps:

1. *Assessment.* Problem areas are selected, specific problem behaviors are selected, the behavior is refined, a contract is agreed on with the client, and such issues as frequency and duration of treatment are discussed.
2. *Verbal instructions.* The therapist provides both general instruction in the procedures to be followed and detailed, relevant verbal instruction to help the client focus on the specific skill to be learned.
3. *Stimulus-modeling tape presentations.* Both the stimulus portion and the responses are presented to the client.
4. *Attention assessment.* The client's reactions to the presentation are discussed. Further, the therapist points out specific stimuli that elicited the model's response.
5. *Focused feedback.* As in standard video replay, the tape is stopped at specific junctures in order to emphasize specific aspects of the situation presented. When presenting a complex task, this stage permits breaking down the task into manageable components.
6. *Behavioral rehearsal.* At this stage roleplays may be used to bolster the learning process or to tailor the situation to the specific needs of the client. These can be videotaped for further feedback.
7. *Performance feedback.* During this stage the client is reinforced for performing the desired behaviors during the behavioral rehearsal stage. If the behavioral rehearsal was videotaped, very specific, focused feedback can be given to the client, and the

client's reactions and feelings about his or her performance can be discussed as well.

8. *Homework.* Specific home assignments, often including behavioral rehearsals, are given to help transfer the learning to the natural environment and to bolster the changes the client has made in his or her repertoire.

These steps are repeated in the above sequence as the client comes closer to achieving the desired goals. The reader will notice that this format, and variations of it, are used in several sections of the book when discussing specific problem situations.

## Movement Therapy

Videotaped replays can add an extra dimension to the movement therapy session. While a client experiences movement activities and exercises largely through a kinetic sense, another sensate experience that is therapeutic in movement therapy is the new way in which a person literally envisions the world while that person engages in unaccustomed forms of movement. A third sensate experience—a person viewing his or her own form—is added through the use of video. This dimension adds a layer of self-confrontation to the movement experience that is bound to be valuable as a way of enhancing how a person gets to know him or herself.

It is beneficial for an individual to watch a videotaped replay of him or herself performing an everyday activity. The group modality allows a person to get to see how he or she relates to others as well, and within a context (creative movement) that is less threatening for some than direct verbal group confrontation.

Incorporating video into movement therapy can be accomplished a number of ways. One may wish to begin a session with a replay of a previous session, or to utilize video feedback solely within the present session. Another alternative is to compare videotapes of previous movement exercises with current ones, and to discuss the changes noticed by the group.

The movement therapist needs a record of movement to function as both a directive and diagnostic tool. Videotape techniques provide a system of recording movement that has many advantages over the two most commonly used forms of record keeping: memory and handwritten notes. Particular exercises can be held for storage and future reference. Cases exemplifying important issues or diagnostic signs, demonstrations for teaching purposes (for both clients and colleagues), or even a movement journal, documenting client change or process, can all be conveniently saved on video.

Video can also be used in conjunction with movement therapy to desensitize people to self-confrontation in general. This can be done by recording only hand or foot movements during a movement therapy session, or by showing hands in the process of creating art objects, gesturing, or writing (McNiff, 1981). This will typically lead to a desire to venture further into self-confrontation, especially when a group member's curiosity is sparked by attempts to figure out whose hands are whose.

Another way of incorporating video feedback into movement therapy is to give group members a printed form that focuses their attention on specific aspects of their own movement. They are asked to notice and briefly comment on the following aspects of their movement:

1. Where are my areas of rigidity? How do I express emotional blocks through these areas?
2. What does the shape of my body tell me about myself? How does the shape of my body interplay with the way I move?
3. How well do I "dance," or interact nonverbally with others? Am I more comfortable with men than women? How do I relate to men differently than I relate to women?
4. Do I move differently around people who are older or younger?
5. What positions do I find particularly stressful or difficult? What does this say about me? Am I afraid of height (upward movement) or depth (downward movement)?
6. What do I notice about myself when the videotape is speeded up or slowed down?
7. Do I need more space around some group members than others? How do I feel about sharing my space?
8. Do I have any eccentric movement habits? What idiosyncratic movements seem uniquely mine?
9. What do I see as I watch myself on video that differs from what I expected to see?

Responses to questions like these help enhance group members' awareness of themselves. Responses can be shared with the rest of the group if a group member feels as though something important was learned. These aspects of communication and expression can also be looked at more informally through discussion led by the therapist.

Certainly, therapists who are attuned to these aspects of the communication process, whether engaging in movement therapy per se or not,
can add an important dimension to their understanding of human
relations.

## The Categories Game

This is a simple group activity adapted from human relations training
for use with video by Gunn (1978). It is a fun activity that allows all
group members to participate in ways that promote group cohesion.

After the videotape recorder is started, the therapist assigns each
group member to a broad category such as plants, dogs, cats, and so on.
After the first group member is given his or her category, the rest of the
group members must quickly think of a specific type of plant, dog, or
cat, for example, that would be appropriate for that individual.
Although everybody is encouraged to participate, it is not necessary for
anyone to explain his or her choice. After each group member has had a
turn, the tape recorder is rewound and replayed. After each client's
segment is played, the tape is stopped and the client is given the
opportunity to talk about his or her reactions to the other group
members' comments, as well as to the general experience of viewing
him or herself on video.

An example of this technique is provided by Gunn (1978, p. 367),
who mentions that when Larry—a loud, independent man—was given
the category "plants," one of the group members responded by saying
"Cactus—hard on the outside, sweet on the inside." Larry described
himself as an artichoke because he had many layers to get through.
Following the viewing of the videotaped replay, the therapist pointed
out to Larry his need to rely heavily on others and his tendency to say
little about himself (based on the comments of the other group
members). These comments surprised Larry, especially since the other
group members so heartily agreed.

## The Outside Therapist

This activity, developed by Gunn (1978), is designed for use with a
group that is cohesive but having trouble addressing itself to specific
group members' difficulties.

Group members are sent in pairs to another room to be videotaped.
One of the two group members is designated "therapist"; this group
member is given a card with an instruction on it. Such an instruction
might read: "Have Jane (the partner) discuss her feelings when her

father left home, and have her show us how sad and angry she was feeling." The "therapist" is instructed to try to gently get the client to disclose his or her feelings, without adding undue stress. The "client" is given the option, as always, not to respond to any prompt that might be too threatening. The interaction between the partners is videotaped for later replay to the group.

As many pairs record these brief segments as time permits. Following this, the segments are played back to the entire group. After each vignette is played the tape is stopped and the group briefly discusses the manner in which the "therapist" performed his or her function. In a sense, the group briefly "supervises" the "therapist," responding to such issues as how sensitive the "therapist" was to the partner's needs. The group also discusses how the "client" responded to the challenge.

Gunn has found that the separation from the remainder of the group, combined with the focused intensity of the video camera, tends to give clients both an added dimension of safety (by being away from the group) and an added amount of pressure (due to the camera's presence). It is hoped that these conditions combine to motivate clients to reveal more about themselves than they would do otherwise. The vignettes that result from this activity provide valuable material for discussion within the group.

# 5

# Group Therapy with Children and Adolescents

The goals of video feedback with groups of children are not much different than those for adults. One hopes to produce a more realistic view of self, a heightened awareness of the way a particular group member relates to another, the identification and change of habitual, self-defeating interaction patterns, an enhanced motivation to change behavior, and an increase in self-esteem.

Video feedback can be an effective intervention with groups of young children. For example, after Noble, Egan, and McDowell (1977) showed video replays to groups of seven-year-old children, the children saw themselves more accurately; they were more conscious of individual differences, physical characteristics, and better able to compare themselves with others. These changes occurred merely by combining simultaneous feedback with delayed feedback of recordings made of the children engaged in free play.

Group therapy with young children must, in my opinion, be either highly structured or unstructured in order to be effective. Highly unstructured groups consist of children engaging in such nonverbal forms of self-expression together as art, music, movement, or play activities. Video can be used here as either a creative tool (that is, as an instrument similar to a paintbrush), or as a passive feedback tool. Highly structured groups usually revolve around either a specific topic which the children discuss or a specific activity, such as many of those discussed in this chapter.

Introducing video to young and latency-age children poses no special problems. In fact, most children jump at the opportunity to play with this sophisticated, alluring toy, and often interest is piqued when the equipment appears in the room. Young children are very familiar with television, typically spending hours of their time in front of their home set. Most children are quite unfamiliar, however, with its ability to recreate one's own experience. An appreciation for the fact that younger children have no idea how on earth a television program comes into being, combined with the fact that many younger children (and emotionally troubled children) do not have the cognitive ability to think abstractly enough to understand the concepts required, will help explain the awe that many children express as the process of viewing themselves on a TV monitor unfolds.

In a group context, children's reactions to seeing themselves on playback are magnified by the ability to directly compare one child's reactions against the other children's. Cowering from one's own reflected image appears more significant in a group in which other children are eager to see what they look like. Avoidant reactions to viewing one's self-image bespeaks very low self-esteem, and it seems not to be the case that this poor self-esteem is restricted to one's physical self-image. In fact, tenaciously avoiding one's self-image is a significant clue to severe depression and pervasive low self-esteem that may not be visible in the typical workings of group therapy.

Groups of adolescents pose different issues. Some typical reactions of adolescents to being videotaped in a group setting are exemplified in the work of Marvit, Lind, and McLaughlin (1974), who attempted to induce attitude changes in 44 delinquent children. The experimental group consisted of 23 adolescents who were videotaped during four group therapy sessions. Following each session, the group members met together to view the tapes and discuss their reactions to seeing themselves.

Initially, when confronted with their own self-defeating behavior, most of the adolescents responded by being more defensive, upset, sensitive, and self-critical than adolescents in groups not using video feedback. The adolescents' positive feelings about themselves diminished as they were less able to deny the effects of their behavior. As their masks of self-confidence gave way to more realistic self-perceptions, the adolescents were more able to discuss their difficulties with other group members. Their vulnerability increased as they became aware of their fears of rejection from others.

But over the four-week group, the responses of the adolescents shifted from negative perspectives of themselves to more positive ones, especially in the important area of physical appearance. This was due largely to the fact that the group members' concern over their appearances led them to dress and groom themselves better. The group members gradually regained positive feelings about themselves, while remaining in greater touch with the self-critical aspects of their personalities.

I have found that less mature adolescents tend to respond initially with a great amount of teasing, and in some cases tremendous self-deprecation. The teasing, of course, is a reflection of discomfort with the technique, the fear of self-exposure inherent in seeing oneself on the monitor. It is a self-protective device that allows the group members to relate in a socially acceptable form which serves to move attention away from the underlying fears of feeling rejected, feeling ugly, and validating self-hatred. It is important that this be interpreted, or at least that the teasing not be permitted to continue, as this will set the stage for avoiding the therapy process throughout the group.

In the early stages of group, adolescent clients may see video as an intrusion, and as a chance to test the therapist's authority. Michel and Blitstein (1979) saw this in action when the two boys operating the video equipment decided to focus exclusively on the therapists' faces. After this initial period, however, group members began to see the video equipment more as a sophisticated toy. At this stage, there was still reluctance to use video as a therapeutic tool. Despite this reluctance, nearly all adolescents enjoyed watching themselves on the screen. This reluctance was greatly reduced after acclimating to the technique.

The therapist should be aware of the possible sources of resistance that clever adolescents may invent. Some may see the opportunity to operate the video equipment as a way to exit the group with grace. Resistance can also be expressed by requesting a video replay in order to avoid the content being discussed at the time. A measure of this resistance is to go ahead and replay the asked-for segment anyway. If group members have difficulty accepting feedback about their behavior, it is a good indication that the group is using feedback in service of resistance. As resistance decreases, group members ask for feedback more appropriately.

Some teenagers respond to seeing themselves on video with severe self-criticism and avoidance. Teenagers who have a propensity to harm themselves and who therefore might use video as a means to validate their self-destructive impulses should be screened out early in the process. Otherwise, it is very important to respond to the individual needs of the adolescent who retreats into severe isolation and self-criticism. Continued self-confrontation, with a great deal of support from the group members, may help depressed adolescents change their views of themselves, but the therapist must remain sensitive to adolescents who are so depressed that they can only see themselves as worthy of dying.

The leader of groups for children and adolescents will find many other activities easily adaptable to this population. Besides some of the activities in Chapter 3 on individual child psychotherapy, the preceding chapter on group therapy with adults offers many activities appropriate for use with children's groups.

## The Activities

### Introductions
In order to get a group of children accustomed to each other, and simultaneously get them acclimated to the presence of a video camera, have the entire group seated in a circle. Each person, in turn, introduces him or herself to the camera while watching the monitor. Each child says hello to the camera and each is encouraged to have a conversation with the monitor. Encourage the child to playfully interact with his or her image, perhaps tell a joke to the monitor, say something about him or herself, exaggerate the person on the screen, move in and out of the frame. Finally, ask each child to introduce the next person. Pass the camera around the circle so that each person photographs the next. This activity can be done without taping (simultaneous feedback), just to get acclimated to the equipment, or it may be recorded and played back. This activity helps children get to know each other without the pressure of directly relating to each other. It is a playful activity that requires interaction in a nonstressful way.

For those children who have difficulty facing their own image on the monitor, the monitor can be hidden from view, and the child can "play around" or have a conversation with the camera lens. This can be replayed later for the child, when he or she has had some time to become a bit more at ease.

### Working Together
This activity is particularly useful for adolescents who have an interest in sports. It can be used as part of an informal discussion group or it can be used in the classroom. If used in a traditional therapy context, it works best in the beginning stages of the group process.

Children are shown a videotape of a team sporting event; basketball games are especially useful for this. After showing segments of the game, stop the tape and review some of the plays. Focus on how the team members worked together to make an important play, and show how a lack of working together prevented certain plays from being made.

The activity is a good forum for discussing issues of individual expression versus fulfillment of group expectations. The therapist may wish to remain in the metaphor or to apply these generalizations to everyday life situations, depending on the therapist's style and the adolescents' readiness.

This activity could easily be combined with video feedback methods in group therapy with adolescents, and the feedback may highlight group processes similar to or different from the teamwork seen earlier. It also may be done effectively in individual therapy with adolescents.

### I Am The Greatest (Talk Show)

This particular variation of the talk show theme has been useful for both latency-age and adolescent children. The therapist functions as the host of a late-night talk show who interviews famous people. The children are asked to write down what they would like to be famous for, since it is necessary that they are famous in order to be asked on the show. The group members are asked to pretend that the show is occurring ten (or more) years into the future, and that by that time they could have accomplished anything they like. Younger children, who may have difficulty with the concept of fame, can be instructed to consider themselves "the greatest" at anything they like. The papers are then collected and given to the host. The videotaping begins with the announcer introducing the host, who then calls up the first guest. While the guest is being interviewed, the remainder of the group serves as the audience. After all the guests have been interviewed, the group gets to watch themselves as they might someday like to be.

This activity serves several purposes. It functions as a vehicle for enhancing self-esteem, helps to clarify goals, and is fun. It also provides a wealth of projective information which could be incorporated later into the group process.

### Script Reading

Reading television scripts is not only an enjoyable experience for most children, but if selected carefully, the scripts can serve to teach children important moral lessons. An example of this was when a group of adolescents read a segment from the TV show *60 Minutes* ("Linda Velzy is Dead") dealing with adolescent runaways and hitchhiking. The videotaping of the script reading enabled the adolescents to watch themselves in the roles portrayed in the script and enhance their identification with the characters. Such script reading, of course, should include a discussion of the content of the material being read.

Scripts can be obtained by writing to the major networks if an adequate explanation of its use is provided. Scripts are also available from several organizations listed in the Appendix.

### At This Point I Feel...

This activity consists of videotaping a group of preadolescent to adolescent children (or older), for approximately one half hour. The group is then shown a replay, but each group member must remain silent until someone shouts out "Stop!" to the operator of the video recorder (usually the therapist). The recorder operator then stops the video (or freezes the action, if equipment allows). The person who interrupts the replay must then make a statement beginning with the words "At this point I felt..." or "At this point I feel...." No comments are made after the person makes his or her statement, thus giving the other group members confidence that they will not be confronted when they make their statements. This permits group members to share with the group feelings they might otherwise be afraid to share.

If a remote-control device is available, it may be placed in the middle of a semicircle. Any group member may then reach over and shut the video off to make their comment.

In introducing this activity the therapist may wish to model for the group members by stopping the tape and making a few comments of his or her own. Group members should be taught to differentiate between a feeling statement and a thought statement. ("At this point I feel like Bobby should shut up" is cheating.) They also should be taught to focus on their feelings in the present ("At this point I feel sad because I miss my brother like John does") or to reflect accurately on their feelings at the time of the group interaction ("At this point I felt angry that John kept talking because I wanted to say something too").

### All That Jazz

An attempt at intermingling a form of music therapy with video feedback was made at the Langley Porter Psychiatric Institute in the late sixties (Wilmer, 1968). A group of drug-involved adolescents was videotaped while simultaneously being shown on a monitor in another room. In the other room a jazz pianist (who also happened to be a psychiatric resident) improvised musical responses to the group's actions while he watched them on the monitor. The music was recorded on a separate track on the videotape, although this was not heard by the group until playback.

When the group members assembled to view themselves on play-back, they didn't like what they heard. Wilmer conjectured that this was chiefly due to the fact that the music made the group painfully aware of their awkward behavior and lack of spontaneity.

Music and video could be combined, however, in a variety of ways, without the necessity of an outside critic. Because music is so much a part of an adolescent's lifestyle, it should prove to be an attractive motivator and therapeutic agent for adolescents. One possibility would be for group members to respond to their own video replays by choosing an instrument (most likely a rhythm instrument, unless a particular group member is skilled at playing another instrument) and "echoing" or "scoring" their own behavior in group while attending to the replay. This could help to increase awareness of an individual's feelings and reactions to other group members, and it can also provide an opportunity for the group to relate together in a manner less threatening than talking.

An alternate strategy would be to videotape the group engaging in an art or dance activity. On replay the group can respond musically by overdubbing the audio channel with its own expression of the feeling being expressed by the group in the videotaped activity.

## Individual Autobiographies

One of the oddities of children's and adolescents' groups, and indeed of groups in general, is how little group members know of each other's outside lives. While this may account for some of the feeling of safety a group provides, it can also be construed as limiting and artificial. Although the group member typically brings to the group his or her individual outside life events, these are distorted through that group member's neuroses; rarely does the group get to see such revealing elements as the individual group member's home, significant others, or the surrounding environment.

In adolescent groups, this can be an extraordinarily interesting and revealing phenomenon. It can be accomplished easily by loaning each group member portable video equipment and encouraging that group member to spend the week prior to the next session recording his or her surroundings or meaningful aspects of his or her life. It can take the format of "a day in the life"—an account of a typical day—or it can take the format of a "photo album"—pictures of those things that the individual finds particularly meaningful or important.

Following the production of the video, the child brings his or her tape to the group and the group reacts and discusses such questions as: "Was there anything in the videotape recording which surprised you?" "How does Joe's life differ from yours?" "What elements do you share in common?" "What feelings that stem from Joe's experience do you share?" "Was there any particular moments that made you feel particularly happy, sad, or angry?"

The therapist should be fairly certain that the group members are supportive enough to give appropriate feedback; if not, this activity could be a terrible experience for the child who bares his or her secrets only to be denigrated in the process.

An alternate way of conducting this exercise is for the therapy group to work "on location" (Reese, 1981). Reese's therapy group wrote and then enacted a script in the actual surroundings at or near where the events in the script were intended to take place. Although Reese's group used super-8 film for this exercise, the technique is certainly adaptable to portable video equipment. The results were telling scenarios of each child's life. Group cohesiveness was evident, and both the therapist and group members learned a tremendous amount about each other's lives and the unique perspectives each brought to them.

The technique also gave the therapist the opportunity to do "on location" therapy. Because the therapist had to drive the group members to several different locations during the course of the shooting, the car became the site for much important discussion.

## Sex in the Other Room

Sexuality is a frequent concern in adolescent groups. While there are a variety of ways of integrating videotapes within a sex therapy framework (see Chapter 8, p. 165), video can provide a route to discussion of sex issues that carries with it a comforting degree of safety.

This can be done by separating the boys and girls to allow for a more comfortable discussion of sexual issues. The girls, for example, can be asked to leave the room while the boys ask questions and discuss various sexual matters (or vice versa). The boys are asked if they mind videotaping this session to be played back to the girls at a later time. Most group members agree to this, and find it easier to discuss sexual issues, even with the knowledge that the discussion will be seen and heard later, without girls in the room at the time of the discussion.

When the girls return to the room (they may have been videotaping their own discussion in the meantime), they watch the replay of the boys' discussion. This can be done either with or without the boys present. Having the boys present relieves their curiosity about the girls' reactions, but it also causes embarrassment; having the other sex gone permits a more open discussion.

This procedure gives the adolescents the opportunity to express empathy, and to see that many of their problems are shared between the sexes. This may help each group discuss their own sexual issues, either within the group at the time, or at a later date (Michel and Blitstein, 1979).

## The Values Game

The game show is a familiar part of most children's lives. This activity combines the excitement of the game show format with a sound values clarification technique, sometimes referred to as the "Values Auction." In the values auction, children have the opportunity to examine their priorities and make decisions about these priorities.

Explain to the group that you have devised a new game show, and that it is called the "values game." You will be the moderator of the show, and you will videotape the show so it can be played back to be discussed later. Give each group member a copy of the "auction list" (an example follows), and $1000 in play money (or any other large, fixed amount of play money). Each child decides for him or herself how the $1000 is to be spent. Each item on the auction list can also be listed individually on index cards for the therapist's use during the game. Explain to the group that you will call out each item on the auction list one by one. After each item is called, group members may bid however much they wish for the item. The item goes to the highest bidder. (You can give the child who received the item the index card with that item printed on it.) The money is handed over before the item is received to enhance realism and prevent cheating. When a child runs out of money he or she can no longer bid.

When the auction is over, the camera is individually shifted to each group member, and the moderator explores with the group members such questions as:

1. What did you receive?
2. Are you happy with what you received?

3. What do you regret not receiving that you wish you could get, and why?
4. Why was a particular item more valuable to one group member than to another?
5. If you could trade one item with another that you didn't receive, what would it be?
6. What are the advantages of having one item (for example, good health) over another (such as money)?
7. Did you feel like you spent your money wisely? Was a particular item so tempting that you blew all your reserves impulsively?

Because this activity can easily take a complete session, play the videotape back during a subsequent session. Use this replay as a "second chance" to discuss conflicts that arose for particular children during the bidding phase. You may wish to stop the videotape at critical points during the bidding and explore what the bidders were thinking and feeling. The choices made will often reflect issues that children express during the course of the group, and these interpretive links are often fruitful to discuss.

Following is an example of an auction list:

1. A free, all expense paid trip to Disneyland, the World Series or a rock concert with anyone of your choice.
2. A chance to spend a day with your favorite TV character.
3. Ten minutes in a store of your choice, collecting whatever you can cart out in a wheel barrow.
4. A perfect backyard, filled with every toy, game or amusement that you can imagine.
5. A guarantee of no war in the world for five years.
6. A guarantee that you will become President of the United States.
7. A week in which no one can tell you what to do.
8. A chance to run your school for a week.
9. A perfect vacation for your parents; they can go wherever they want and do whatever they want for a week, at no cost to them or to you.
10. Perfect health for your entire life.
11. A chance to become the most beautiful or most handsome person in the state.
12. The opportunity to eat whatever you want for one year.
13. The chance to personally solve the world's pollution and environmental problems.

14. The promise to have a perfect friendship for life; your friend will be exactly what you want him or her to be.
15. The promise to become a rock or country music star.

## Six O'clock News

In the six o'clock news, children play TV newscasters. The heart of this activity is the roving reporter who interviews children (and staff, in inpatient settings) about their feelings and opinions concerning issues relevant to them. The questions may be generated by the therapist or by the group members. When played back to the remainder of the group, the therapist may wish to stop the tape at junctures that may lead to therapeutic clarification and discussion.

Issues for discussion may be political in nature, or they may be personal. The personal questions may involve asking children for their opinions about hot topics such as premarital sex, involvement in drugs, or the effects of divorce on children. For younger children, personal questions may more appropriately revolve around what it feels like to be left out of a group, not chosen for a team until last, teased by a sibling or classmate.

Although this activity provides an important outlet for discussion of pressing topics, beginning with less threatening questions may help children to feel comfortable discussing more personal issues later. Less threatening questions may be in order for children who are particularly sensitive to discussing their feelings. In this case, the reporter may ask such questions as: "What do you like best about school?" "What is your favorite thing to do at home?" "What is your favorite TV show?" "What would you do if you had a hundred dollars?" "Describe a 'perfect day' for you." "If you were the leader of the group, how would you lead it differently?" "What is your favorite sport?" "What kinds of things are you good at?"

Although these questions may not deal with deep conflicts, the responses help children to define their self-concepts more clearly, and therefore to feel special. The support and interaction of the group, the feeling of mutuality in coming to see that others share one's intimate values and opinions, the support and positive regard of the therapist, and the clarification of individual values are the main therapeutic ingredients of this activity.

## Learning from Soaps

Soap operas are tailormade vehicles for discussion of the most volatile and sensitive issues which confront each of us. They are display cases into the conflicts that touch many of our lives, and certainly nearly all of our imaginations. For those who believe strongly in "values clarification" and "moral education," soap operas provide high-octane fuel for discussion of personal values and societal mores. Elements of soap operas exist in nearly all households, and discussion of segments of soap operas can provide an entryway into the world of the child's home, a world the child may have been reluctant to discuss in group without a safe vehicle.

This activity is simple, but it requires some preparation. The therapist records a soap opera and then selects those segments which may be appropriate for discussion. These carefully selected segments are then played to the group members who are asked to discuss what they think is going on in the segment. "What could have preceded this short vignette, and what do you think will follow it?" "What do you believe *should* follow it?" "What would you do if you were in so-and-so's shoes?" "Have any of these events occurred in your home?" "How did you feel when they did?"

The therapist should feel ready to drop the showing of a preplanned segment in order to follow the needs of the group members at the time. The purpose of this activity is to stimulate group interaction and discussion; rigid adherence to a preplanned structure could blind the therapist to subtle cues that could potentially move the group closer to dealing with relevant therapeutic issues.

## Commercials for Myself

This highly structured group activity is excellent for younger children, especially those in an institutionalized setting where many children's self-esteem is compromised by virtue of the feelings and cognitions associated with being set apart from other children.

This activity is best begun by discussing the purpose and concept of advertising to the children. Have the children watch some pre-recorded commercials. In discussing advertising, emphasize the reason for selling products to other people, and that good advertising not only convinces but informs people of what makes the product unique and special. Tell the children that in this activity they are going to be the product, and they are going to try to sell themselves to others as people who would make good friends to others.

These commercials can be made during group, or after group on the children's own time (if the children are in an inpatient setting). Completed commercials are then shown to the group and discussed. Discussion generally centers on what makes each child special. Other children should be encouraged to add anything they can think of to the list of characteristics chosen by the student. Competition among the children for making the best commercial should be discouraged, while emphasis should be placed on each child's unique qualities.

## Video Interviews

This activity is particularly useful for children in inpatient settings for it requires the production of videotaped interviews outside of group times. It can also be used, however, in day treatment settings as a classroom activity. The production of videotaped interviews is an indirect but highly effective way of teaching children interpersonal skills. Because the elements of effective interviewing parallel the elements of effective communication in general, the therapist who "coaches" interviewing skills can do much to indirectly enhance interpersonal skills, and hence self-esteem, among his or her clients.

The skills that an effective interviewer should learn include the following:

1. Preparing the subject. Try to relax the subject who you wish to interview. Be aware of personal space; sit or stand at a distance that is comfortable for the subject. Engage the subject in light conversation before the interview.
2. Asking questions. Focus on the "here and now." Use questions the subject can identify with from his or her own experience. Try to avoid "yes" or "no" questions, so that you have the opportunity to help the subject rephrase his or her responses. Don't dominate the interview. Be patient, honest, and respect privacy.
3. Listening skills. Show interest by maintaining good eye contact. Concentrate on the person's response, and not the next question.
4. Summarize at the end of the interview.
5. Express gratitude to subjects for their participation.

These skills can be taught by the therapist or day treatment teacher to the children who may also be given a printed list of the above items. Furthermore, interviews can be rehearsed or roleplayed within the group, with video feedback following with the above items serving as a guideline for feedback.

Children should also be given topics for an interview, and they should choose an appropriate person to interview. This may be a staff psychiatrist, janitor, technician, nurse, psychologist, or clerical worker. The following topics may be used for assignments:

1. What does it take to become a nurse (psychologist, secretary, and so on)?
2. What do you think a psychologically "healthy" person is like? How are people transformed from feeling down in the dumps to feeling good?
3. Interview handicapped people. Talk about fears, feelings, problems of coping with handicaps.
4. What sex roles and family stereotypes do people assume? Who should do the dishes? Who should do the household repairs?
5. Interview a relative as if you knew nothing about this person. Find out about this relative's past, his or her likes and dislikes.
6. Interview people from different countries or different cultures. What kinds of struggles do they endure?
7. Choose a question from an advice column. Interview people who have different opinions about the question.

The video interview process is one that builds self-esteem because children create products they are proud of and that are uniquely theirs. Furthermore, it permits children to interact with people who they otherwise might not notice, using the camera and the interview assignment as the legitimizer of the social interaction.

### Let's Put an End to All This

Pre-record a television program—either a drama, comedy, or movie. Play this program back to the group, stopping after various points of conflict. Ask the children how they think the program will end or how the conflict will be resolved. Explore various alternative endings and resolutions to the conflicts.

This simple activity has the effect of increasing children's awareness of alternative ways of solving their problems. Children will learn strategies from other group members as well as from the therapist. It will also promote thinking through conflicts and will model problem-solving approaches to problems. This is accomplished by the therapist encouraging the students to follow their line of reasoning out to its logical conclusion, and by occasionally modeling problem-solving strategies for the group members, thus decreasing impulsive acting-out.

## Dream Sequence

This activity is appropriate for older, more sophisticated children. Have the group members record their dreams into a dream journal. Attempt to relate exactly what occurred in the dream. Take a particular dream or dream sequence and evaluate it for how well it may be translated into a video production. Allow each group member to develop a script from his or her dream sequence and have the child create a videotaped "dream." The child assigns parts to the other group members, rehearses briefly, and then records the final version. Children should be forewarned that their production will not, nor need it, accurately reflect the dream.

Encourage discussion following the viewing of each dream. Discuss the nature of symbolism and metaphor, ways in which one thing may represent something else. Emphasize the personal, individualized nature of symbolism, and refrain from overinterpreting a person's dream. Encourage the person who created the videotape, however, to freely discuss possible interpretations. Also discuss with the group members their feelings about the roles they were playing.

It will become clear that the group members may not wish to resolve the dream in the same way the child's dream was resolved. This gives the therapist the opportunity to explore alternative resolutions.

## TV Excerpts

The showing of excerpts from television commercials or other programs can be used therapeutically in a number of ways. What follows are a few simple, structured uses of TV excerpts in group therapy with children.

*Portrayals.* Television commercials are notoriously offensive in their stereotyping of sex roles. Videotape several commercials and show them to the group. Discuss traditional sex roles as they are exemplified in the characters on TV. Use this as a springboard for a general discussion of the effects of sex role stereotyping on our individual and cultural values, and on feelings of self-worth.

Discuss the portrayal of handicapped people on television, as well as the concept of being handicapped. Broaden this to a discussion of people's fallibilities and general strengths and weaknesses. Discuss the notion of compensation. Also discuss how it feels to be the butt of condescending jokes. Why do people make fun of handicapped people? Discuss this in terms of people's fears of being handicapped themselves and how people often turn their fears into scapegoating.

Television excerpts can also be used to discus cultural and socio-economic similarities and differences.

***Hidden Messages.***    An excellent way to teach children to be sensitive to underlying meanings, and thus to improve their communicative abilities and deepen their understanding of themselves, is through the concepts of overt and covert messages. These are difficult concepts, and require a high level of cognitive functioning.

Discuss the fact that most messages have at least two levels, the overt and the covert. Give group members examples of everyday messages, like "I had a great day today. My teacher gave me a note that said I did all my work in class." Point out that the covert message might be "I want you to be proud of me, and tell me that you care about me." Have the group members come up with overt messages, to which you supply possible covert interpretations.

Television excerpts, especially commercials, can be excellent media for exploring these concepts. Present group members with a TV commercial and ask what they think the overt message is. After obtaining the fact that the overt message is to buy the product, ask what the covert, or hidden messages are. Help the students by giving examples, such as the underlying message about the role of men and women in society, the underlying message about the importance of winning in sports, the underlying messages about how people ought to behave in certain situations, and so on.

***Persuasion.***    TV commercials, and advertising in general, are good modalities for teaching children communication skills. This can be done by examining the techniques of persuasion used in advertising. View some TV commercials and have the students point out when they believe one of the following techniques is being used:

Bandwagon: "Everybody's doing it."
Repetition: Saying or showing the product repeatedly.
Use of emotional words: Choice of words intended to elicit strong
    feelings.
Testimonial: A famous person saying, "I use this product."
Transfer: "If you use this product, you will be like the happy and
    exciting people we are showing you."

This exercise can be expanded by having children make their own commercials using these techniques, or by having them try to sell an idea using these techniques to the remainder of the group. It may also be combined with "Commercials for Myself" (p. 88).

***Future Schlock.***   This technique is used to help assist children who may have difficulty separating fact from fancy. Tape record a science fiction program such as an old "Star Trek" repeat. For young children you may wish to use cartoons. View the program with the group, stopping occasionally to ask whether certain things could really happen today. For example, you may ask whether someone can be "beamed up" to a space ship from a planet. You may ask if there really is such a thing as a Vulcan. To make the game more fun, be sure to include things that are possible. Is it possible to have such a large TV screen to see what's going on outside a spaceship?

This activity is not intended to rob children of their fantasies, which may in fact be healthy fantasies. The exercise should be done only with children who tend to confuse their fantasies with their realities. These children will find relief in knowing that "The Incredible Hulk" is not real.

## Turn That Thing Down!

The purpose of this activity is to elicit and discuss feeling through the use of television music. Because television music is designed specifically for this purpose, it lends itself extremely well to a discussion of the use of sound to elicit feelings. Choose a show with a good musical background; a frightening movie is excellent for this. Demonstrate the importance of music in creating a mood by showing segments of the TV show without sound. Have group members try to guess what kind of sound should accompany the scene they are seeing. When a frightening moment seems imminent, turn off the sound. Demonstrate how the scary effect is diminished by turning off the sound.

By turning the contrast knob to black on the video monitor or TV set, the sound can be played without the video image. Try to find moments when sound is used to heighten apprehension or to elicit lilting, happy feelings, or sad, morose feelings. It is also fruitful to focus the children on drawing connections between the scene they are viewing and the music they are hearing. Discuss the rationale for choosing a particular type of music. This entails a discussion of the scene that is occurring and the contextual variables that pull for particular feelings. This helps the children to develop a greater sensitivity to their feelings and the feelings of others, as well as to the situations in life that typically arouse certain feelings.

## Hey, What's Your Angle?

The art of cinematography and photography in general encompasses a psychology of its own. Photographers use different angles and shots to elicit different responses from the audience. For example, close-ups imply intimacy and perhaps confrontation, while long-shots imply distance, perhaps independence and solitude. Shots taken from below eye level, looking up at a subject, communicate superiority and power, while shots taken looking down upon the subject communicate inferiority and weakness. Shots taken from a side angle may indicate dubiousness, that is, "looking askance."

In the group, have the children develop scenes which are intended to communicate seeing someone in a certain emotional light. Then have group members use the camera angles above to create the atmosphere in a short videotape. Play the videotapes back to the group and discuss the feelings they elicit.

You may wish to videotape a scene from a variety of different angles as a demonstration to the group of the way in which different angles evoke different feelings. You may also have the students watch a segment of a television show and identify the kind of shots the director chose to use. Discuss why the director may have chosen a particular shot in light of the kind of feeling the director wanted to elicit in the audience. Discuss how it feels to have to look up to people or look down on them. How does it feel to be close to someone? How close can you get without feeling frightened? What does it mean to look askance at someone?

## Space Case

The activities in this section are experiential methods of learning the importance of personal space. Aspects of these activities are in part based on those presented by Kaplan (1980) and Travis (1977). The first method is more appropriate for younger children while the second requires the sophistication of adolescents.

Mark off a square on the floor to serve as an imaginary elevator. Start the videotape recorder running and call each child individually to stand inside the square. Don't tell them, however, that the square represents an elevator. Fill the square up with group members, but do not overcrowd the square to the point at which group members have difficulty remaining inside.

When the square has been filled, stop the videotape and have the group seated. Replay the videotape, and discuss your and the children's observations. Discuss where the initial person stood in the square, and where the second person stood in relation to the first. What does this say about personal space? What happened as more and more people entered the square, and what were their feelings as they felt their territories shrink? What happens to arms and legs as more people enter the square?

Now repeat the activity once more, telling the group that the square is really an elevator in a crowded department store just before closing time on Christmas Eve. Let the children choose props, if available, and have them roleplay entering and exiting this crowded elevator. Replay the videotape, and discuss the group members' feelings now. What did they notice on the replay about eye contact? Where should people look when they are in a confined place?

This activity could lead into a fruitful discussion concerning the need to have a place of one's own. The therapist might wish to have group members attempt to recall situations in their lives when their personal space was violated, such as a sibling moving into the child's bedroom or fights about who gets to sit in the front seat of a car. You may wish to bring up topics such as territoriality at the dinner table and in the group, or the relationship between territoriality and feelings of possessiveness and self-esteem.

The second activity deals more directly with sociological and political concerns. Discuss with the group what would happen if there were five or six times as many people in the group as there are at present. Delineate a small space of the room and call it the universe. Turn on the videotape recorder, and fill that small space with the whole group and one chair. The task of the group is to negotiate for space and comfort. It may be necessary to convene and record a World Council with individuals representing different planets and different ideologies. Have the group members prepare and present proposals; negotiate agreements concerning boundaries, space travel, immigration, energy sources, and peace and security arrangements.

Replay the video and discuss the issues that emerged, focusing not only on the feelings of security and trust, or lack of it, in individual members. Use the videotape replay to display revealing facial expressions when the children are cramped into a small space. Discuss also the need for depending on others for security, and how it feels to be dependent on others. Discuss how these needs are threatened when space is confined, or when food or comfort is withdrawn. These issues can be related to specific issues being discussed in the group, or specifically to issues related to certain group members' family lives.

# 6
# Family Therapy

Communication theorists have given psychotherapists a strong foundation for understanding complex family systems. One aspect of communication theory particularly useful to family therapists is the notion that people communicate with one another via communication channels and that these channels can frequently portray different messages, some of which may be contradictory or incongruent. Videotape methodology provides an excellent way of bringing conflicting messages to the awareness of clients because of its ability to repeatedly examine communication patterns. This awareness is often encouraging and reassuring to both the sender of the message and the recipient. Senders can discover the reason they get the kinds of reactions they do, and recipients are reassured that they aren't crazy and truly do pick up a particularly confusing message. It is important to recognize that a certain degree of "double-binding" behavior in families is healthy; it can be the breeding ground for creativity, humor, and the ability to accept the ambiguity inherent in life. However, pervasive, restrictive double-binding behavior that serves to keep the family system in a pathogenic or homeostatically uncomfortable, unrewarding, unhappy cycle, can be the breeding ground for severe pathology.

Satir, Stachowiak, and Taschman (1975) see videotape as providing a self-portrait based on the Sartrean metaphor of one's life being a self-portrait consisting only of that which an individual has become. Satir shows families videotapes of themselves, asks them to rate what they see, and to then respond with a list of those things about themselves that they would like to change. The fact that the videotape can be erased repeatedly provides another metaphor for the therapist; over the course of therapy the self-portrait can be continually replaced with a new one. Satir videotapes a family at different junctures in therapy in order to show them their changing portraits.

The "second-chance phenomenon" was discussed by Alger and Hogan (1967a). This relates to the notion that because there are multiple channels of communication, and because video permits repeated replays of an event, attention can be focused on a particular channel of communication that might have been missed the first or second time around. Thus, one marital partner might discover a nonverbal behavior contradicting a verbal behavior that could not have been seen without a second chance.

Videotape also permits an increased objectivity in family members as they examine their own behavior. Through replays, the therapist provides the family or the couple with a "truthful" reflection of their interrelationships. This truthfulness is often a dire need in families who are experiencing extreme discord (Silk, 1972).

In couples therapy, video replays reinforce the modeling that occurs by the third person when a therapist interacts with one of the partners. For example, the therapist's helpful, supportive attitude in dealing with one partner's difficulties on playback serves as a model and a reinforcer for the other partner (Nadelson, Bessuk, Hopps, & Boutelle, 1977).

One of the chief roles of the family therapist is to point out significant repetitive family patterns. Through repeated viewing of replays it is easy to sensitize family members to their patterns; under such circumstances the therapist need only give a brief cue in order for a family member to recognize the particular pattern being played out in the replay.

Berger (1978) highlights some of the typical repetitive family patterns that can be easily seen in video replays. These include the placating pattern ("Yes, you're right, you're always right"); the blaming pattern ("Whenever I do that it's your fault because ... "); preaching ("When I was younger ... "); changing the subject; withdrawing; denying; somatizing; discounting; and finally, being mature and realistic.

The distressingly common blaming pattern is one that many family therapists (for example, Alger & Hogan, 1967a; Kagan, Krathwohl, & Miller, 1963) have isolated in connection with video feedback; these therapists report that clients are more willing to take responsibility for their own part in creating a dysfunctional relationship after viewing video playbacks. Many of the above patterns can best be identified by such nonverbal cues as when a family member dismisses another with the wave of a hand, thus continually discounting that family member. Video replays can also be used to reinforce a therapeutic breakthrough at a later time during the course of treatment (Bodin, 1969).

Through examination of video feedback, alliances between family members can be seen much more clearly. Clues to this include coenesis, or interactional synchrony, in which one family member moves in rhythmic synchrony with another. These synchronicities often occur without the participants' awareness, but nevertheless indicate salient alliances. Likewise, distance or animosity among family members can be seen in turning away from a particular member or putting up a nonverbal blockade, such as legs crossed as if to shield another family member. Also, shifts in family alliances can be easily detected through repeated examination of nonverbal behavior.

It is often helpful, after the first video feedback session of a family, to keep in mind the possibility that one family member's nonverbal behavior may be an icon for the entire family. A father's grim countenance may bespeak a lifeless family, uniformly victimized and helpless.

Within a cybernetic model of family therapy, video interventions can be seen as providing negative feedback, that is, feedback that discourages the family's "stable instability" and promotes the development of a more functional homeostasis (Alger, 1973). The therapist introduces interpretations of behaviors, the purpose of which may be seen differently—completely and tenaciously—by a family member.

Whitaker (1978) points out that because family rituals have been refined for generations, the therapist's unique and lucid vision is more easily clouded in family therapy than it is in either individual or group therapy. Thus, Whitaker has found that videotape helps him to be more objective about his own subjectivity, and that videotape feedback helps to divert him from "mothering" the family. Whitaker also sees video as a way of breaking through difficult therapeutic impasses, especially useful if a consultant or co-therapist is unavilable.

Some family therapists believe that it is often desirable for the therapist to be seen as an equal partner in the therapy process (Alger & Hogan, 1969). Watching video replays fosters this equality because video replay entails a mutual exploration of both therapist and client behaviors, and because in video neither the observing therapist nor the client can change the behavior already fixed on the screen. The effect of this is greater personal involvement for the client, and greater willingness to change. The mutual exploration of therapist and client allows family members to feel as though they have discovered their own behavior without the therapist pointing it out.

As with group therapy it is often valuable to allow different family members to act as camera operator, thus permitting a view of the family from that member's unique perspective. Allowing a certain family member to operate the camera also helps that person develop an increased sensitivity to nonverbal behavior and to the nuances that may set off patterned behavior.

## The Activities

The activities in this chapter deal with the use of video in either couples or family therapy. The sections on parent training and sex therapy found in Chapter 8 (pp. 160 and 165) may also be relevant to a family therapy context.

### The Serial Argument

The family sits in a semicircle with the camera facing the family from the open end of the circle. This permits the individual videotaping of each family member as he or she talks. The family, or the therapist, decides on a topic for a family argument. This should probably be a topic with which the family currently has difficulty. The family is instructed to act as they would in any family argument, with two important differences. Each family member will speak in turn and say no more than one or two sentences at a time. The family continues until either a resolution to the argument comes about, or until the therapist, sensing that a resolution is not about to occur, decides to end this portion of the activity.

The videotape is then played back and stopped after each family member says his or her one or two sentences. The therapist may wish to offer an interpretation at this point or to further question the family members in order to explore the motivations for particular statements. Family members may wish to comment on seeing themselves or to discuss such things as how they felt when they were speaking, how they felt when another family member spoke, or what sort of roles may have emerged.

Following this, the therapist may wish to direct the family to argue serially again, or the therapist may wish to have the family freely discuss the argued topic once again. This final stage of the activity can occur with or without videotape. A videotaped playback of this portion, however, may help to reinforce the new insights or different ways of behaving that the family may have learned during the first feedback portion of the activity.

## Family Roleplay

At the beginning of a session, the family is instructed to choose an episode of importance to them that occurred during the past week. They then roleplay the incident, playing themselves, attempting to stay as close as possible to what actually occurred. The entire roleplay is videotaped and played back. During the replay any member can stop the machine at any time and reflect on his or her own behavior or the behavior of other family members. During this time, discrepancies in recall inevitably occur. It is best at this point to avoid discussing these discrepancies unless, in the therapist's judgment, a problem arises that is serious enough to warrant interrupting the flow of this technique.

After viewing the replay, the family members are asked to repeat the episode, this time incorporating anything they may have learned from viewing the roleplay or listening to the discussion. The revision is videotaped and then played back in its entirety without stopping for feedback. Once more the family is asked to play out the episode, this time more spontaneously as they feel they would like it to occur at the moment. It is during this final version that resolutions to old difficulties are often discovered by the family, even without the intervention of the therapist.

The family roleplay was pioneered by Alger (1973), who believes that it helps change the roles of the therapist and family members. Alger believes that during the replay both family members and therapist become "data researchers," equally involved in reviewing and reacting to the videotaped material. Alger sees this as fostering a healthy mutuality between clients and therapist, a mutuality that helps to make psychotherapy a more human adventure.

The family role-play technique can be productively altered by the addition of such traditional role-play adjuncts as role reversal or role switching, in which one family member takes on the role of another. Techniques used in psychodrama (see Chapter 4) can also enhance this activity.

## Family Sculpture

This technique is an adaptation for video of an activity initially used by Satir and her colleagues (1975). Family members take turns sculpting a scenario representative of their feelings about the interrelationships within the family. Each family member is instructed to construct a scene, using any props available, representative of the ideal family. The remaining family members are all considered props as well, and they can each be put into position by the family member constructing the scene. The entire process is videotaped.

After the first family member is finished constructing his or her ideal family, that same person is asked to construct a scene portraying his or her real family. The sculptor is asked to try to place the family in positions indicative of how they typically behave toward one another.

After all family members have completed sculpting their conceptions of their ideal and real families, the videotape is reviewed and discussed by the family. Discussion inevitably centers on the reasons for making certain choices. When a person is seen to be indecisive, it is important to clarify what conflicts were occurring for that person at the time. When a person initially places one family member in a certain position and then changes it, discussion might reveal what insights the family member had at the time. Discrepancies between real and ideal concepts of family, as well as discrepancies among family members in their portrayals of these concepts, serve as fertile ground for family discussion.

## Three Covert Messages

This is a method of peeling away layers of defensiveness in order to increase self-knowledge. Because it is done with a partner, it also increases a couple's knowledge of each other, and in so doing it helps to improve communication between them. While this technique may be performed in the therapist's office with the therapist's help and guidance, it can also be performed at home by any couple with access to video recording devices.

The couple is asked to discuss anything they like for ten minutes. The topic should be something meaningful to both, but it need not be a major point of contention. A small disagreement serves best because it avoids the highly emotionally charged issues that may interfere with the successful completion of this activity.

The ten minute interchange is videotaped. No single partner should be permitted to dominate the discussion. A rule that keeps the discussion simple may be employed: Each person should speak no more than a few sentences before the other person responds.

After ten minutes the discussion is stopped, regardless of whether or not there is any closure to the discussion. The videotape is replayed but stopped after each comment. After listening to each comment, the person who made that comment is required to "peel three layers off" that comment. Peeling a layer means that the person is to try to get in touch with the covert message underlying the overt message spoken. Covert messages underly every message and may be very simple, but they are by their nature hidden from awareness at the time they are spoken. A person who may have difficulty accessing the other things that were on his or her mind at the time may wish to merely fantasize what other things may have been on his or her mind at the time. The person who is not "peeling" must not comment during or immediately after his or her partner gives the three covert messages. Such judgmental comments as "I don't believe you were really thinking that," or help, for example, "I think you really were thinking . . . " must especially be avoided. The players alternate back and forth, giving three covert messages after each comment. Partners should be encouraged to use their nonverbal appearance on the screen to discover their covert messages.

The activity ends when both partners agree that they have had enough. If the rules are followed closely, this can be an enormously therapeutic and valuable learning experience for both partners.

An example of a dialogue that might emerge follows:

*Playback.*

HE: Well, I think I'd like to talk about the cat, about the fact that I think I'm kind of annoyed that you haven't done anything about making an appointment to get the cat spayed. (*The tape is stopped.*)

HE: Well, the first covert thing is that I realize that I've been wanting to bring this up for a long time, and I guess I'm a little annoyed at myself that I didn't bring it up sooner. I guess the second covert thing is pretty obvious, and I can tell from my expression that I'm pretty disappointed in you and that I'm holding back some anger. I can see the anger in my eyebrows. The third thing . . . God, this is hard. I'm not sure, but I think there's a part of me that simply wanted your attention.

*Playback.*

SHE: I didn't know I was the one that was supposed to make the appointment.

SHE: That was sarcastic of course. Except I really didn't know I was the one who was supposed to make the appointment. [Comment: This is a rule violation; this time period should focus only on covert messages underlying what was presented on the videotape. No new material should be introduced here.] The first covert message is that I guess I was pretty pissed off. I felt like you were manipulating me the way you always do. The second covert message is that I wish you wouldn't manipulate me, and the third covert message is . . . well, I wonder, maybe I was supposed to make the appointment, and I forgot all about it.

*Playback.*
HE: Well, I don't think we ever really agreed that you were the one who was supposed to make the appointment, but you were the one who was bugging me about this for about a month, and if you really cared about it I figure you'd do something about it. (*The tape is stopped.*)
HE: The first thing is that I have a feeling when I watch this now that at the time it really wasn't the cat thing that was bothering me. That must be an example of something a bit deeper. I'm not sure what that is. The second thing is . . . well, I guess that is a bit manipulative, but I really wasn't aware of it at the time. The second thing is . . . maybe I was just annoyed that you never seem to do anything on time—you're really a procrastinator, and you don't seem to pay attention to the things you should. The third thing is, well, I don't know, but maybe one of the things I felt like you procrastinated about was me. Maybe I didn't feel like you paid enough attention to me.

*Playback.*
SHE: So what's the big deal? If you wanted me to make the appointment, I'll make the appointment. Why didn't you remind me? (*The tape is stopped*).
SHE: I'm still angry, although I'm still not really being straight about my anger. Maybe that's why my anger always builds up to the point where it explodes. Anyway, the second covert message is that I think I wish you weren't so nasty all the time. I feel like you always get angry at me about little things. The third thing is that . . . I don't know, I can't really think of a third thing. (Long pause.) I think when it was happening I was slightly aware of the fact that I was being a little manipulative too, and I feel guilty about that.

## Cross-confrontation
Paul (1968) has developed a family therapy procedure called "cross-confrontation," in which a family views provocative segments of another family's videotapes. This activity requires consent from the "donor family" to use the family's videotapes in therapy sessions with other families. This must be sensitively and carefully explored with the family; extreme care must be taken to not violate the privacy of the family whose tape will be seen by others. There are different opinions

among professionals regarding the ethics of such a procedure. It is my view that, although significant therapeutic value is often obtained through the therapist's allegiance to strict confidentiality (which should always be honored unless the client specifically gives uncoerced permission to violate this principle), this confidentiality can also give the client the message that being in therapy is something to be ashamed of. In fact, it may breed a pathology orientation to the therapeutic process which runs counter to my own feeling that the self-rating inherent in seeing oneself as sick is a fundamental problem; it usually serves only to validate poor self-concepts and self-hatred. By presenting the family with the philosophy that they are basically just as healthy (or unhealthy) as any other family, it is much less likely that the family will refuse to permit the therapist's discretionary use of its videotaped segments. One way of avoiding this problem altogether is to use well-acted roleplays of intense family interactions.

The purposes of the cross-confrontation procedure are manifold. The therapist may wish to use the segments to motivate the recipient family to discuss significant issues which it might have difficulty discussing due to shame, guilt, or one of a variety of forms of resistance. Confrontation with another family's therapy may be used to show the recipient family members that they are not alone and that they can be helped as much as have other families. Perhaps the most significant use of the tapes is as models to demonstrate how to work through difficult therapeutic impasses. Another important use is as a prompt or provocateur to provoke the family into discussing issues that it had avoided.

The response to this form of confrontation varies tremendously, from completely denying the videotape's relevance to overt, empathic identification with the donor family.

In preparing the cross-confrontation tapes, it is important to edit out only those segments that might apply to the family who will be watching the tape. Brief, relevant segments serve to decrease resistance in that it is less likely that families will be disinterested or that their attention might be distracted by irrelevant stimuli.

## Multiple Family Therapy

In multiple family therapy, five or six families are brought together to discuss difficulties and to problem solve (Laqueur, 1973). The therapist is the conductor of the 20 to 25 people assembled; he or she typically works with a co-therapist, observers (trainees), video camera

operators, and supervisors. These sessions are conducted in a large
room where approximately 30 chairs are placed in a circle or
semicircle.

Video is used primarily to enhance the family members' awareness of
nonverbal messages communicated within this large group. The groups
are loosely structured; the therapist usually begins by asking if the
group wishes to begin a new topic or to continue discussing something
mentioned at a previous meeting. After the group talks for a while, the
therapist attempts to find a common theme. After 15 to 20 minutes, the
therapist will often break up the discussion by asking a question such
as, "Shall we review what we have done so far?" This review can then
be accomplished by replaying the videotape of the beginning of the
group for the families. The group members then watch and comment on
their behavior and interactions, thus preparing them for a more active
and intimate description and examination of their attitudes and
feelings.

Video is also used by Laqueur as a way of interrupting families who
tend to monopolize the group. By calling for a replay, the therapist
encourages other families to join in and interfere with the monopoli-
zation.

An alternative is to structure the use of video more carefully. After
several sessions of building trust and rapport, the therapist identifies a
particular issue on which a family may work. This issue should be one
that many of the families share. The family is then called on to roleplay
this issue, in a manner similar to that mentioned in "Family Roleplay."
This roleplay is videotaped and replayed to the entire group who add
their own perspectives, including supportive comments, criticisms, and
suggestions.

## Filial Therapy

Filial therapy is an approach to child psychotherapy in which parents
are taught to be therapeutic agents for their children (Guerney, 1964).
Parents are seen in groups in which they are taught to conduct play
sessions within carefully delineated guidelines. Hornsby and
Appelbaum (1978) modified the technique to provide more direct
training of individual families utilizing video feedback as part of the
training modality.

Hornsby and Appelbaum note that this technique is particularly
successful with hyperkinetic, withdrawing, or overanxious children,
who maintain an active conflict with one or both parents. The positive
aspects of the relationship can be reinforced and the conflict areas can

be quickly exposed. The technique is not as effective, however, for dealing with severely neurotic children who have deeply internalized conflicts, children with significant personality disorders, or psychotic children.

The program begins with the parents and child evaluated both separately and together with an eye toward assessing the degree of conflict between the child and each of the parents. The parent who seems to relate to the child in the least conflicted way is given the title of "primary therapist." This parent is then given a rundown of the procedures to follow, which includes conducting weekly, half-hour play sessions in a well-equipped playroom. While the sessions are being conducted, both the professional and the other parent watch through a one-way mirror. The parent is kept in touch with the others in the observation room through the use of a small, battery-operated hearing-aid device called a "bug-in-the-ear." During the session the professional can make comments and/or give instructions to the primary therapist, as well as give a running commentary to the other parent. Furthermore, the play sessions are also videotaped. The procedures are also clearly explained to the child who is not deceived in any way.

After each session, the parents are seen together by the professional for one half-hour parent therapy session. The parents discuss their feelings and observations about the session, and the videotape is played and reviewed. A specific focus is placed on the communication patterns that exist between the primary therapist and the child. Discussion typically moves from concern over technique to exploration of feelings and problems relating to the child.

The technique is an attempt to recreate aspects of the parent-child interaction in the controlled setting of the playroom. When ineffective ways of relating are seen, the professional has a way of helping the parent deal with these feelings as they occur, as well as an opportunity to reinforce this learning following the session.

## On Again/Off Again

This activity turns an ordinary on/off switch into a technique. The concept for this activity is derived from Bodin (1969), who recommends using the on/off switch, which is often available in remote control form, as a way of reinforcing desired behavior and punishing undesired behavior. The therapist essentially doles out approval or disapproval by his or her choice of what to videotape and what not to videotape.

One example of the use of this method is having the therapist switch off the recorder in the midst of the verbose, controlling, pedantic father's diatribe to his daughter. In general, a therapist who sees a particularly maladaptive interaction pattern might announce this to the family. The therapist then says that he or she would like to get it down on videotape in order to study the pattern later. From then on, each time the therapist turns on the remote control switch, the family members wonder what they have done to warrant special attention. If the therapist wishes, special focus can be placed on an individual family member; if so the therapist may wish to make his or her reasons for focusing on a particular family member clear prior to acting on these wishes. This buffers against family members misconstruing the therapist's reasons for such a special focus. The therapist may later wish to announce a change in this focus.

Bodin believes that this procedure may, in the long run, prove less distracting than continued verbal interruptions from the therapist reminding family members of their dysfunctional communication patterns. The procedure also pressures the family to monitor its own behavior, which also decreases the likelihood of the therapist using interpretations to disrupt the family system.

While it is true that a variety of disapproval signals occur constantly throughout the therapy session, the use of the switch helps make the therapist more aware of how and when to intentionally put those signals to use.

After a while, the on/off switch can be offered to any member of the family. A family member may wish to use the switch to demonstrate a particularly offensive behavior of another family member. Struggles over who gets to use the switch provide potentially useful process material. Bodin notes that the wish to escape being caught by another family member may provide a strong incentive to change.

## The Role Game

The illumination of specific roles that people take can be an extremely productive venture in family therapy. Berger (1978) has listed some of the more common roles individual family members play: jester; referee-umpire; catalyst; Don Juan; the idiot; injustice collector; the abused type; missionary; crisis creator; storyteller; clock-watcher; whiner; leader of the opposition; nitpicker; self-righteous critic; expert; provocateur; fragile baby; general; intellectual; flirt; sophisticate; troublemaker; monopolizer; charmer; iconoclast; victim; vindicator; frail tyrant; prosecutor; seducer; scapegoat; rejection collector; saint; innocent; advice seeker; virtuously honest sadist; overprotective mama;

the doctor's assistant; martyr; ombudsman-guardian; negativistic clique creator; help-rejecting complainer; runt of the litter; strong silent type; can't say no; manipulator; competitor; ostrich; fair one; Pollyanna; castrator; guilt provoker. (p. 193)

There are a variety of ways these roles can be incorporated into family therapy. In general, the therapist should be on the lookout for these roles as they emerge in the video replay. Identify the roles by name for the client, and then replay the section of the videotape in which the family member is playing the role until he or she understands it.

Alternately, place each of these roles on an index card. In order to help family members become aware of roles, have them choose a role from the deck at random and play that role in a family discussion. Replay the videotape and have family members guess which roles each other were playing.

Another variation is to have each family member choose appropriate roles for the other family members. The cards are then given to the family members; they are to portray these roles as they discuss an issue. The video is replayed and the roles are discussed.

## Stimulus-response Sequences

This procedure is somewhat unwieldy; although it is complex and time-consuming, it does present an interesting and potentially highly productive way of ascertaining areas of difficulty among family members and of stimulating family discussion concerning these relevant issues. The framework for this procedure was provided in a research context by Goldstein, Judd, Rodnick, Alkire, and Gould (1968), and although video was used to provide feedback, audiotape was used through much of the actual technique itself. Shifting to videotape requires some extra work; both methods are beneficial, but the videotape adds realism and seems to increase motivation and active participation. Because of the complexity of the technique, it is recommended for use only with triads—two parents and a child or two children and a parent. Furthermore, many variations of the technique are possible, and it is recommended that the clinician tailor this technique to his or her own time exigencies.

The first step is to see each family member separately. Each family member is given a standardized interview in which seven areas of adolescent–parent conflict are explored. These include achievement, sociability, responsibility, communication, response to frustration, autonomy, and sex and dating. Each of these areas is discussed at length in order to isolate conflicts that are limited in scope and specifically germane to the particular family.

After isolating the conflicts, the therapist asks the individual family members to roleplay a specific example of the problem as if the family member were talking to the other person in the conflict. The family member is told to try to bring the other family member around to his or her way of thinking. Following the roleplay, family members are asked to predict as closely as possible the response of the person to whom the convincing arguments were directed. The prediction is called an "expectancy," while the argumentative statements are called "cues." Both the cues and expectancies are videotaped, enacted as if the other person were in the room. Both parents separately generate a set of cues for the child, and the child generates a different set for both parents. (The child, therefore, generates two sets of cue statements.)

Next, in a separate individual session, the intended recipient hears the cue statements made by the other family members directed at him or her. After hearing each cue statement, the family member responds to the message as if the person were present. This response is also recorded. The end result is a series of stimulus roleplays given by one family member and the responses made to those roleplays by the other family member.

This procedure may be varied somewhat by including presentation of the same cue statement to the respondent, but this time the respondent hears the other family member's expectancy statement next and is then played the cue statement one more time. After hearing both the expectancy and cue statements, the listener responds to the cue statement. It is interesting here to see if the listener intentionally shifts away (or toward) the expected response.

Following the taping of the cue–response sequences, family members are brought together in the confrontation phase. In dyads, family members are asked to talk about one of the problems to which they have just reacted in the simulated interaction portion of the session. The relevant tape segment is played to foster the interaction. The members of the dyad are asked to talk about the recorded sequence, including the reasons each responded in the manner he or she did. They are then asked to attempt to resolve the issue in a way that is satisfactory to both. A total of five minutes is allotted for dyadic discussion of each issue.

This procedure results in each dyad discussing two problems—one in which the cue was directed from the child to the parent, and the other in which the direction was reversed. After discussion of the two problems, the parent is removed from the room, and the other parent is brought in to undergo the same sequence of events. Next, the third family member enters the room and three-way interaction sequences (dealing with two different cue–response sequences) take place. Seven minutes are allotted here for discussion.

Notably, family members are left alone during these confrontation sequences. These sequences, by the way, are also recorded on videotape. The fifth session utilizes the tape made of the confrontation phase for purposes of video feedback. Here, the stimulus-response sequences and videotapes made of the confrontation phase are used to stimulate further discussion among family members, this time in a more open-ended, exploratory fashion.

This technique, although complex and highly structured, results in family discussions that are highly realistic and that deal with important family issues.

# 7

# Training and Supervision

Prior to the widespread use of audiotapes in supervision, students could only bring to their supervisors remembrances of their previous encounters with their clients—remembrances easily distorted through the various defensive filters that defined each student's personality. At best, student therapists had to rely on notes taken during the session; these notes were, by their nature, intrusive and not immune to subjective filtration. The supervisor's hypotheses about the nature of the therapist–client interaction were necessarily based on the less than optimal data base of the therapist's selective memory.

Audio techniques are a vast improvement over this inefficient and often ineffective method of supervision. The supervisor is given a more direct sense of how the therapist actually acts in the therapy session. Audio permits the supervisor to listen to a therapy session in its entirety, and allows him or her the freedom to select portions at will. But audio also gives a distorted picture of the therapist–client interaction, for it prevents access to the crucial nonverbal messages available to the student therapist at the time of the session.

The importance of nonverbal behavior, including gestures, body movements, facial expression, and paralanguage, should not be underestimated. This often denied aspect of communication provides innumerable keys to the covert messages and feelings of both client and therapist. In dealing with children who communicate predominantly through nonverbal channels, videotape replays are essential. In such cases in which progress is measured in small units as with a highly regressed adult or with an autistic child, a smile and a headnod in response to an intervention may be a crucial bit of information. It is common for beginning students to neglect nonverbal cues, slowing the development of the crucial third ear, or ability to understand the client's unintended yet significant meanings.

Two alternatives to supervision by notes or by review of audiotapes remain: observation of the therapy session through a one-way mirror, and having the supervisor sit in with the therapist during a therapy session. When using the one-way mirror, observers must sit in dark, small, and often poorly ventilated rooms, conducive to weariness and inattentiveness. Furthermore, one-way mirrors are not completely soundproof, so that discussion of a case while viewing it is hampered. The chief problem with the supervisor sitting in on a session is that it changes the nature of the therapeutic relationship and may feel intrusive to the therapist and to the client.

In most forms of supervision, the supervisor never actually sees the client. According to Chodoff (1972), this has two possibly deleterious effects. First, it deprives the supervisor of a great deal of information about the client, and second, it may cause the supervisor to focus undue attention on the trainee to the neglect of the client and the client's welfare. Video makes it easy to see and get to know the client, giving the supervisor access to important aspects of behavior that may have been overlooked by the student, and causing the supervisor to focus a more balanced amount of attention on the client. These factors tend to combine to cause a larger investment by the supervisor in the actual treatment of the client.

Another important aspect for the supervisor considering the use of video is that it tends to facilitate a professional distance; this is due to the fact that once an event is recorded on tape, it is fixed in the past tense and is, therefore, unchangeable. The physical framing of the picture in an artificial box also contributes to this distancing effect (Evans & Clifford, 1976). Furthermore, videotape reduces some of the speculation that often removes supervision from the events in the actual session; if there is uncertainty in the recall of a particular event, one can return to the replay and find certainty.

The supervisor using video should make use of video's ability to help both novice and experienced therapists to improve their subtle communication skills and to enhance self-awareness. The inaccurate timing, small gestures, use of jargon, and lack of spontaneity which tend to escape consciousness at the time of the event do not escape the unrelenting replay. By the same token, videotape also permits the therapist to see him or herself being witty, clever, intelligent and incisive. For better or worse, video will help fantasied images of one's therapeutic stance give way to a more accurate picture.

Another important aspect of which supervisors should remain aware is the fact that it is less likely that the student therapist will consciously screen remembrances of the session from the supervisor. This fortuitous aspect occurs because most everything about the therapist–client relationship is out in the open; it is therefore difficult for students to act out the conflicts they may have with their supervisors within the therapy session (Chodoff, 1972).

As a teaching tool, video reinforces what is typically only heard or read with what is seen. This addition of a visual sense cannot be underestimated as a reinforcer of learning. By providing learning programs through commercial television, or in making tapes available to the public for home viewing, learning can occur in the home where there is not only privacy but also an environment where much of the learning can directly transfer. Students who have difficulty learning can view videotapes privately, at their leisure, as can students who are unable to attend classes or demonstrations. Videotapes can be accessed by therapists during cancellations and no-shows.

Video is an extraordinarily flexible tool for both teaching and supervision. It can be stopped and started at will, permitting the supervisor and supervisee to spend as much time on a particular aspect of the therapy process as they desire. The videotape can be run for long periods of time without interruption, giving a more global sense of the course of the session. When a pattern is noted it can be reviewed, or a return to an earlier part of the tape may indicate the root of a certain turn in the session. Missed interventions can be noted as well.

Through the use of close-up or zoom lenses personal space can be invaded without the discomfort arising from moving one's chair up close to a client (Forrest, Ryan, Glavin, & Merritt, 1974). As a teaching tool, there are certain procedures that lend themselves to close-up work. Nurses, for example, can be taught catheterizations and injections easily through the use of close-up video recording.

Images or demonstrations can be multiplied to allow the display of information at two or more physically separated locations. This permits instruction to a large audience either in a single lecture hall on several monitors or through the viewing of demonstrations potentially channeled into hundreds of rooms or offices where viewers can participate in the comfort of familiar surroundings. Other technical advantages of video include the abilities to superimpose one image on another and to utilize split-screen techniques.

The large quantity of information collected by video is a prominent problem inherent in the use of video in supervision. Because of this large quantity of data, it is important to limit what is used and commented on when viewing the replay. It is easy to miss the forest for the trees and become so concerned with minutiae that the overall strategy of the therapeutic encounter becomes obscured (Chodoff, 1972). The supervisor must resist the temptation to comment every few moments, despite the irresistible and often blatant opportunities to make brilliant remarks.

Perhaps one of the most unfortunate problems with videotape in training is that it will not transform a poor supervisor into a good one. In fact, it probably will expose the supervisor's weaknesses, as well as highlight his or her strengths. A willingness to expose one's own clinical experiences to students will provide valuable modeling for students and will also give students the opportunity to see if the supervisor practices what he or she preaches (Wilmer, 1967). Those supervisors who are uncomfortable with their own therapeutic skills or those who find themselves disappointingly rigid or embarrassingly inappropriate would do better with some other form of supervision. Because videotape playback is incapable of selective attention, therapists must be prepared for the discomfort involved in such self-exposure. Knowledge of this discomfort is a vital source of empathy with those students who risk similar self-exposure.

The use of video will likewise not make a good teacher out of a bad one. Without enthusiasm, interest, and ingenuity, most audiovisual presentations will be as appealing as uncarbonated soda. Roeske (1978) pointed out that audiovisual materials have a remarkably ambivalent position in learning. Because television is so familiar, students are attracted and accustomed to it as a learning device. Yet because of years of poor programming and ridiculous commercials, most students also learned well how to selectively tune out uninteresting materials.

In both supervision and teaching, video should not be used exclusively. Its greatest utility is in dealing with the details of interaction processes. Overuse of video will tire the student and the supervisee and will lessen the likelihood that students will be able to cope with more global, abstract forms of knowledge. The best way to handle video is to intersperse it with conventional uses. Schiff and

Reivich (1964) recommended "spot monitoring," in which video is used on occasion to supplement traditional supervision. In teaching, the challenge for the educator is to develop the most effectively stimulating and judicious blend of a variety of learning materials and experiences.

Although video provides a great amount of information, it still reduces the amount of information derived from a live interview. There are nuances perceived by the therapist in the live interview that often cannot be detected on the video replay. The degree to which the expression of emotion on videotape is accurately communicated is open to question. There is, of course, something missing from a televised portrayal of feeling when compared to the live experience. The intensity of a brief moment of silence, the discomfort inherent in a barely audible sigh, all seem understated on video. The television monitor has a way of smoothing over intense moments. Certainly, it is more difficult to feel empathic with a video image than it is to feel empathic in a live situation. Video is best used in supervision as a way of stimulating the therapist to new insights, reviewing patterns, and finding sources of specific reactions; it cannot replace the intuitive processes and spontaneity born from the tension of the live encounter.

Some supervisors and students who have not used video express concern over the reaction of clients. Typically, the vast majority of clients participate readily, are not stressed by the experience, barely notice the equipment after a brief period of acclimation, and are willing to take part repeatedly (Schmidt & Messner, 1977). Even when psychiatric patients were videotaped via closed-circuit television for teaching purposes to a large number of students, most patients enthusiastically rated the experience as positive (Barnes & Pilowsky, 1969).

The experience of videotaping is usually much more anxiety provoking for the student. At times, complaints about the video equipment or the mechanics of the procedure can mask students' fears about their competence as therapists. Supervisors can help this situation by not overidentifying with the students' anxieties, by nondefensively introducing video to students, by legitimizing and discussing students' fears, and by sharing their own tribulations with using video in therapy. Roleplaying the introduction of video to clients can also help allay students' fears (Schnarch, 1981).

The supervisory meeting may begin with a discussion of the session from the student's perspective, thus giving the student the feeling that his or her feelings will be respected. Such an endeavor might in fact lead the supervisor to deciding it is best not to view the videotape at all. The student is best involved in the videotape review process as a collaborator.

Other difficulties in either the supervisory relationship or the primary therapeutic relationship can be expressed by the student "forgetting" tapes, showing only "good" tapes, or being continually embarrassed. Schnarch points out that at these times it is often wise to focus on the therapist's feelings toward the client and/or the supervisor and the effect those feelings may have on treatment.

The varieties of video applications for supervision and training are substantial. Video is used in training psychologists, psychiatrists, social workers, marriage and family counselors, nurses (see for example, Hector, 1970); pharmacists (see Love, Henson, Wiese, & Parker, 1979; Mutchie, Bosso, & Higbee, 1981; Schwinghammer, 1981); music and art therapists (Greenfield, 1978; Alley, 1980; Hanser & Furman, 1980); crisis intervention workers (Folsom & Grant, 1978); and teachers (Fuller & Manning, 1973). Video has also been used beneficially in the training of teaching skills (Bazuin and Yonke, 1980).

Besides those listed in this chapter, many techniques in this book may be adapted for use in training and supervision. "Half and Half," "Freeze!" "Serial Viewing," "Speed Shift," "Interpersonal Process Recall," and "The Split-screen Technique" are especially valuable techniques for training purposes.

## The Activities

### Group Supervision

The most common use of videotaped therapy sessions in group supervision entails playing back the videotape of a supervisee's therapy session to the remaining students in the group and permitting any member of the group to call for a halt and perhaps a replay at any point in the tape (Adler, Ware, & Enelow, 1970). This can be a very threatening process for the novice therapist. One method of decreasing defensiveness is to give the first exclusive opportunity to comment about the replay to the student therapist who is under scrutiny (Katz, 1975). The student, carefully facilitated by the supervisor, is invited to relate his or her feelings about the session. Other group members should be permitted to add their reactions, but the supervisor may request at the outset that direct criticism be avoided. Other ways of alleviating some of the tension include: the supervisor may set the stage by initially presenting a videotape of his or her own work for self-scrutiny and scrutiny by the group; he or she may discuss sources of resistance that may be felt by group members; and the supervisor may be certain to give balanced feedback.

The following strategy may be advisable with a group that is more advanced or more comfortable with self-analysis. The supervisor stops the tape at a chosen point and asks each group member to state his or her opinion as to how to proceed. Each group member is also asked to predict what might occur when the videotape playback is resumed (Chodoff, 1972). Each week a different supervisee presents a case and the process is repeated. (If possible, group supervision should immediately follow the session that was videotaped. This capitalizes on increased recall of the subtleties of the interaction not apparent in the videotape replay, and allows the supervisee to benefit from timely reinforcement.)

One advantage of this technique is that not only does each member of the group receive the input of every other member of the group but also each trainee receives the benefit of learning from a variety of different clients. This method also encourages group members to take an active role in the supervision process and tends to awaken even the sleepiest participant. Another advantage is that it gives the student who is being observed the opportunity to hear the variety of different and acceptable approaches that may be taken with a case. This in turn helps trainees to understand the important notion that there is no one correct way to conduct psychotherapy. It also permits students to hear different theoretical perspectives that colleagues may bring to the group.

The supervisor's role becomes more passive when the remainder of the supervision group becomes active and more capable of making supportive comments. The supervisor, then, can focus more on drawing connections between ostensibly different viewpoints, and on summing up statements made by the group.

A disadvantage of this technique is that it can be more stressful for trainees than most other approaches to supervision. After all, the therapist-in-training now has to worry about criticism from both the supervisor and the peers who compose the remainder of the supervision group. The supervisor must remain sensitive to this fact and must interpret supervisees' discomfort and defensive maneuvers. Furthermore, students may find that they don't look as good on video replays as they sound when they personally relay information about their sessions. This may be due to students' overestimation of their clinical acumen, and it may also be due to the added tension (for both the student and the client) inherent in the video situation.

## The Continuous Case Conference

The continuous case conference differs only slightly from group supervision mentioned above. Usually, case conferences focus more on coming to a better understanding of a client than on specifically improving the psychotherapeutic or diagnostic skills of the primary caregiver. In the Department of Psychiatry at UCLA, a monthly continuous case conference is held in conjunction with supervision (Gruenberg & Liston, 1978). At the conference, a wide range of treatment personnel gather to discuss a single patient who is selected for presentation for the entire year. Segments of representative portions of the videotapes of the resident's sessions are shown at this case conference, and the participants discuss their reaction to the patient, the resident, and their ideas regarding treatment. The leadership of the conference is shared between the supervisor and visiting consultants. Both the presence of the visiting consultants and the diverse helping professionals give the resident and the participants the opportunity to incorporate variegated treatment strategies.

Similar continuous case conferences are held at the University of Nebraska (Benschoter, Wittson, & Ingham, 1965), and at a multitude of hospitals and clinics throughout the country.

When presenting a client for the first time, it may be advisable to use segments of ten to fifteen minutes in order to orient the conference participants. Longer segments may be needed to illustrate themes. Brief segments are best used if there is a question of whether or not a particular behavior did or did not occur (Schnarch, 1981).

Videotaped presentations of clients may also be useful in grand rounds conferences. Instead of using the standard live interview, a videotape is made of the patient prior to the grand rounds meeting. A variety of important details, including important diagnostic characteristics and defense mechanisms, can be elicited, recorded, and later edited so that a representative portion can be presented at the meeting. This prevents the frequent problem of obtaining only minimal information from the client at the time of the conference due to the brief time allotted for the patient interview.

This procedure also eliminates the occasional embarrassment patients feel when they are exhibited before a large group. Those patients who may be easily distracted by a live audience, for example, psychotic patients and children and adolescents, may be benefited by this less obtrusive procedure. If the presentation involves an outpatient, this procedure makes it unnecessary to schedule the patient for an "on call" appearance (Suess, 1966).

## The Live Interview

The live interview also represents an attempt at altering some of the offensive aspects of the grand rounds procedure. This procedure, developed in 1958 by Dr. Raymond Waggoner, involves interviewing patients privately while simultaneously presenting this interview over closed-circuit television to a group of professionals (Holmes, 1961). It also includes the use of an audio intercom between the person teaching the group of professionals and the interviewer (Holmes, 1961).

A selected client is interviewed in a studio while a group of students observe monitors of the transmitted interview in a large auditorium. On a technical note, it is often distracting to have too many monitors visible to any one student. Fewer monitors (or perhaps the use of a large screen), along with an explicit instruction to the audience to restrict attention to a single monitor, help to prevent lapses of attention. The lecturer remains in the auditorium but maintains contact with the interviewer through the use of an intercom.

As in all videotape procedures outlined in this book, the client is made fully aware of the entire procedure before participating. The client is asked for consent to be videotaped on closed-circuit television. Closed-circuit is explained briefly. The client is then told that the interview will be seen by a large group (in my opinion, the client should be told the number of people observing) of clinicians or students who are interested in learning about the kind of problems and difficulties the client is having, in the hope that it will do something toward making them better clinicians. The client is not told that the observers are "interested in you and want to help you"; this will go further in unsettling client trust than will the truth. The client should also be told about the physical arrangement of the studio and the intercom system between the teacher and the interviewer. In general, the client should be made to feel as free as possible to decline the request without apology.

The interview itself should be oriented toward history taking and current symptomatology. Potentially embarrassing information should be avoided. If, during the interview, the interviewer receives a question from the lecturer over the intercom earphone, the client should be directly told of it. Besides being difficult to do otherwise (because it disrupts the interviewer's train of thought), an attempt to hide these questions justifies an increase in the client's suspicions.

The live interview technique permits simultaneous close-up observation of a client by many students; it therefore allows greater teaching economy without undue sacrifice of respect for the client's comfort—a sacrifice that may be great under the pressure to perform directly in front of an auditorium filled with clinicians. The use of a current client gives the audience a sense of immediacy and credibility in excess of that obtained by the use of an edited videotape of a session that may have occurred a long time ago. Videotape recording may still be applied during the live interview, especially if the client being interviewed presents unusual or important features.

On the other hand, the use of a live interview may make it difficult to demonstrate what the instructor or interviewer wishes to demonstrate, especially because many clients dramatically improve under the pressure of being examined before a television camera. Because of the unpredictable spontaneity that occurs during the live interview, the lecturer cannot easily resort to canned clinical descriptions or theoretical abstractions. The lecturer must instead respond to the challenge of real clinical circumstance, and the students' demands for clarity and concreteness.

## Group-splitting

Kaufman and McElhose (1973) devised a useful exercise in their attempt to train dormitory resident advisors in group counseling issues using videotape methods. A group of resident advisers was split into two groups. One group went into an adjoining room with a leader; their task was simply to interact in an unstructured manner, while being videotaped. The second group remained in an observation room and observed the first group via closed-circuit TV. Members of both groups were told that following the interaction–observation session they would regroup as a whole and rehash what had occurred in the interaction group. This rehash period was also videotaped.

When the members of the first group—the interaction group—met, they discussed what they were interested in achieving from the training experience, while the members of the observation group attempted to discern significant issues emerging from the interaction group. The leader of the group provided information on group psychodynamics in order to increase the group members' awareness of what they were seeing. The rehash period seemed to be the most potent aspect of this training exercise. The observers did much to help the interactors see their own dynamics.

In the second session both groups and group leaders changed roles. The new observing group was now competitive and eager to find flaws in order to prove that they were doing the better job. The rehash period then became the laboratory for the group dynamics which were being acted out between the two groups. Because the rehash period was also being videotaped, the group leaders were able to play back segments in which the two groups were avoiding dealing with significant issues.

In the third session the two groups were brought together for a videotaped session. Initially the separate group identities were still clear, although gradually these barriers were crossed and a fertile exchange of feelings ensued. Disappointment, anger, and a genuine desire to communicate became apparent, and at the end of the third session the whole group seemed to coalesce.

Seven more sessions followed, in which videotape was not used as an adjunct. The authors attribute the use of videotape to an increased ability to confront many feelings which otherwise would have taken much longer to reach. Combined with group splitting, intense feelings of anger and competitiveness arose early, as did the mutual need to resolve these feelings. This then led to a much more cohesive group which was able to use its confrontational experience as a solid base from which to understand group processes and eventually, to feel comfortable leading groups under supervision.

This group-splitting technique can be a powerful technique for training any helping professional—therapist, counselor, teacher, or nurse—in group dynamics and in helping people to sensitize themselves to their own impact on others. The combination of didactic and experiential learning inherent in this activity is common to most of the activities to be found in this chapter and forms the essential core of the training of mental health clinicians.

## Student as Supervisor

A supervisor is a unique blend of teacher (one who transmits knowledge), educator (one who transmits wisdom), and therapist (one who heals and guides). It is the challenge of every supervisor to motivate students to take an active, inquiring part in the business of seeking knowledge, wisdom, and personal growth. Barchilon, as quoted in Berger (1978), developed a unique system for motivating students to take more interest in the process of learning about doing therapy. His proposition was simple; students will be more involved and active when given the opportunity to take the role of supervisor, that is, to switch roles with the supervisor. The system works in the following manner: First, students watch a videotaped therapy session of the supervisor in the role of therapist with an actual client. This occurs without the supervisor present. Then students take the role of supervisor, with the intent of criticizing and teaching the therapist. At first students will ease their discomfort by offering mostly praise to their teacher, but if the teacher can remain nondefensive, this will soon change as students gain confidence. The therapist/teacher must try to consider the truth in the students' criticisms and maintain an attitude of passive acceptance, despite the students' increasing tendency to project onto the teacher a wide range of their own transference reactions. If the therapist becomes defensive, the students are likely to revert to their accustomed position of subservient passivity.

In this form of supervision, the supervisor must expect rather excessive hostility due to the fact that a student's stored anger at being "one-down" as a student throughout his or her life finally has a chance to surface. This hostility, manifested in hypercriticism, may last about three months until the next stage emerges. This next stage consists of a strong identification with the therapist/supervisor. As the therapy parallel continues, students eventually resolve their ambivalent identification and move into an attitude of realistic cooperation with the supervisor. This final stage is one that facilitates perspicacious observations of processes occurring within the session.

Barchilon found that this technique worked remarkably well even with students who did not appear to be either psychologically sophisticated or initially sensitive to their own or others' feelings. The technique is especially useful for undermining resistance and antagonism in the reluctant student.

## Intake/Evaluation

Many hospitals and clinics utilize video in the intake and evaluation process. Because it is often inappropriate for large numbers of people to be obtrusively observing or participating in an intake, it is a common procedure to use a closed-circuit system to observe the intake in another room. With proper consent, the intake can be recorded and played back for use as part of the diagnostic evaluation process or even as part of the treatment process. The evaluation process can of course be continued with the videotaping of play sessions or structured interviews.

Not only do these initial videotapes provide information valuable to the assessment process but they also serve as sources of useful baseline data with which later videotapes can be compared as a measure of therapeutic progress.

## Closed-circuit Collaboration

When a medical center in an urban setting wishes to carry on an affiliation with a hospital located in a remote area, or when a consortium of clinics wishes to maintain contact with each other for educational purposes, closed-circuit television transmission may provide an economically and extremely useful solution.

These video connections can be made available through arrangement with the local telephone company which can provide transmission channels for two-way audio, video, and intercom service. Arrangements can also be made with telephone company officials to assure that these transmissions can be kept completely confidential.

One of the many examples of a long-distance link is the two-way system between the Nebraska Psychiatric Institute, located in Omaha, and Norfolk State Hospital in Norfolk, Nebraska, 112 miles away. This system began operating in 1964 and has been used extensively in inservice training of hospital personnel involved with the care of patients. The grand rounds held weekly at the psychiatric institute are transmitted to the staff at the state hospital, and they participate through their two-way connection. Likewise, occasional rounds emanating from the hospital are transmitted to the institute. (Benschoter, Wittson, & Ingham, 1965)

Another application improves diagnosis and treatment of patients at the hospital. Through the video connection, long-distance consultation on issues of treatment and diagnosis is available in instances in which distance would have otherwise prohibited such an arrangement. Specialized services, often unavilable to remote state hospitals, can be made available through the video connection. An example of this is speech therapy; it has been demonstrated that speech disorders can be evaluated via television, and in some cases, speech therapy can be conducted via a two-way television system. (Benschoter, Wittson, & Ingham, 1965)

One of the most important applications of the video connection is that it permits the use of the resources of the state hospital for teaching purposes at the psychiatric institute. The hospital provides a larger variety of psychological and psychiatric disorders than would be available to the institute. Therefore, interviews with interesting cases can be presented to the institute which can then be presented to students at the institute either immediately or saved in videotape form to be shown later. Notably, the combined videotape libraries (see p. 134) of the hospital and the institute can be made available immediately through the two-way connection.

Other uses to which the two-way video system in Nebraska has been applied include:

1. securing information about a patient's illness from family members in the Omaha area;
2. working with individual family members when distance prevents them from coming to the hospital;
3. in the conduct of family therapy;
4. to "visit" with the patient over long distances;
5. follow-up and counseling after placement in a vocational rehabilitation program located in an urban area;
6. collaboration on joint research ventures;
7. presentation of a research seminar to state hospital staff.

## Inservice Training

This is perhaps one of the oldest uses of videotapes. Pre-recorded videotapes can be used effectively as teaching tapes for psychiatric residents, psychology interns, special education teachers, and nursing students in a multitude of ways. One of these is to expose trainees to such issues as the intricacies of diagnostics, behavior modification strategies, conflict resolution techniques, interviewing and dynamics as they arise during psychotherapy sessions. Lectures of guest speakers may be presented, and guest speakers may use videotapes to demonstrate specialized procedures or to present examples of their therapeutic work. Not only will this serve to didactically teach students new techniques but it will also provide valuable modeling experiences for students. If videotapes are presented by staff members, students are given the opportunity to see if the teacher practices what he or she preaches (Wilmer, 1967).

## Supra-supervision

Goin, Kline, and Zimmerman (1978) developed a simple, non-threatening method for involving supervisors in the task of learning how to better supervise. Psychiatric supervisors were invited to watch and talk about videotapes of supervisors who were rated by residents as being excellent teachers of psychotherapy. As measured by both the residents' assessment of their supervisors and the supervisors' reactions to the process, this method proved to be effective in enhancing several important supervision skills. It is an intrinsically interesting technique for supervisors, for it allows observing supervisors to yield to their voyeuristic urges while not risking exposure themselves.

Goin and colleagues made two 45-minute videotapes; each tape was composed of three 15-minute segments demonstrating the supervision of three highly ranked supervisors. The 15-minute segments were obtained by carefully editing representative portions of one hour's worth of supervision. One tape was discussed per meeting. After watching each quarter-hour segment, the tape was stopped and discussed by the supervisors. At this point, supervisors were asked what qualities the videotaped supervisor had that might have led that supervisor to be highly regarded by the residents. Qualities the supra-supervisors had in common were also discussed. It was necessary to instruct the group of supervisors to concentrate on positive feedback to curtail a tendency to criticize aspects of the supervision.

The results of a well-designed evaluation concluded that exposing supervisors to a videotape of excellent supervisor–resident sessions changed their behavior. Residents saw them as significantly more active in helping them to synthesize client's psychodynamics, in understanding psychotherapeutic technique, and in gaining a theoretical understanding of the therapeutic process. The newly trained supervisors also directed more attention to areas the residents had not considered while more frequently pointing out mistakes and talking about countertransference.

While one of the advantages of this technique is that supervisors do not have to subject themselves to the strain of being videotaped themselves and are therefore less resistant, it is important that supervisors who supervise others with videotape at least get an idea of what it feels like to be videotaped themselves. One method for obtaining this is for the supervisors to videotape their own supervision sessions and replay these either for self-evaluation or for replay among colleagues who are willing to discuss and criticize each other's supervisory skills. Besides the fact that this is an excellent way to improve one's supervision skills (and thereby to indirectly improve client care), it also sets a positive model for the trainees who appreciate the fact that their supervisors are undergoing a parallel process.

## The Composite Videotape
The major goal in this technique is the creation of a useful tool to aid in the training of clinical supervisors. The technique calls for making a composite videotape consisting of segments of a supervisee's therapy session interspliced with relevant portions of a supervision session.

The therapist and his or her supervisor together review a videotape recording of the therapist's therapy session. With either of the two stopping the videotape when warranted, alternative therapeutic strategies are explored. This discussion is also videotaped. The videotape of the supervision session is then combined with the tape of the therapy session so that the supervisor's comments immediately follow the relevant portion of the therapy session.

This final tape is then viewed by members of a supervision workshop or team that consists of a mixture of students and faculty or clinic staff. The main focus of this meeting is on the supervisory technique, although it is unavoidable that some aspects of the actual psycho-therapy will be discussed.

This "supervision of supervision" technique was employed by Watters, Elder, Smith, & Cleghorn (1971) at McMaster University with great success. Supervisors, unused to being observed or criticized, felt as though they improved their supervisory skills, while interns felt better equipped to utilize supervision because of their overall involve-ment in the learning process and because they became clearer as to both supervisory technique and the goals of the supervisory process.

## Microcounseling

Microcounseling is a paradigm for training counseling skills that was originated by Ivey (1971; Ivey & Authier, 1978). Because it focuses on highly specific skills, it is particularly amenable to assistance with video methods. Microcounseling reduces interviewing skills to individual components that are mastered serially and finally combined into a complete performance. The components include eye contact, posture, listening, prompting, and paraphrasing. These components are seen as necessary (but not sufficient) to learn in order to become an effective therapist or counselor.

Videotape is used to provide students with models that demonstrate each of these component skills. Students then roleplay, emphasizing the acquisition of the particular skill under study. These roleplays are also videotaped and used as a source of feedback. Students repeat the role-play feedback loop until they reach criterion performance levels.

The particular skills that comprise this format are mentioned briefly in the section on parent training in Chapter 8. Detailed strategies for teaching these skills are outlined in Ivey and Authier (1978). The microcounseling format is useful in a variety of different sorts of training, including family and group therapy. It is useful in teaching supervision and in consulting with businesses.

## The Scrapbook

Just as clients can benefit from seeing their growth in therapy over time, so can therapists-in-training. An example of this approach might be called the video scrapbook because it contains brief samples of therapists' work as it accumulates over time. Wilmer (1968) developed this idea at the Langley Porter Neuropsychiatric Institute. There, ten-minute samples of first-year residents' initial interviews were video-taped. The taping continued at six-month intervals so at the end of the three-year residency, residents accumulated video scrapbooks of their growth while at the institute.

## Pre-course Taping

An interesting combination of videotape and live demonstrations was developed by Dr. Sheldon Starr of the Mental Research Institute for use in training family therapists (see Bodin, 1969). The technique calls for "pre-taping" a family's initial therapy session approximately one month before the first class session. The videotape is played and discussed during the first class session, thereby creating a way of noting changes which occur by the time of the family's fifth session. The fifth session occurs just in time for the second week of class, which is a live demonstration of the same family for the class. This simple procedure permits a short-term class to see changes which actually occur over a longer period of time than the class has available.

Depending on the length of the course, subsequent demonstrations could continue, giving the students a greater sense of the typical pace of family therapy sessions. Live demonstrations or videotaped sessions of other families may be interspersed for the sake of variety, usually without much risk of students' losing the ability to maintain interest in the primary family.

Pre-course taping is especially valuable for teaching short courses, for example, a two- or three-week family therapy workshop.

## Doing It Yourself

Although the professionally produced, mass-distributed videotape can be an extremely valuable aid to teaching, there are drawbacks. First, it may be difficult to find a videotape suited precisely to your own needs, especially if you are teaching a course in an esoteric area. Second, many videotapes that are available commercially are out of date.

To remedy these difficulties, you may wish to produce a videotape yourself. If you are not trained in television production methods, however, you should be aware of the enormous undertaking required to produce a television program of professional quality. Such an undertaking, besides requiring a large investment of time and money, realistically requires the expertise of a production company or at least of a trained director who knows the entailments and has the technical skill to accomplish such a mission.

Collaboration between mental health professionals and television production professionals can be rewarding and fruitful. Assuming that the production crew will handle the technical details, here are some things you should be prepared for from your end of the deal:

1. Know your subject. Whatever you decide to be the topic of your presentation, you will be expected to be familiar with the latest knowledge about that topic. If you are producing something that will utilize guest speakers or experts, you must know who they are and how to get them. If you are writing the show yourself, you will probably need to interview the experts beforehand. Knowing your subject also requires knowing your slant, or your approach to the subject. You should have a unique or refreshing slant if your topic is one that can be read about elsewhere. Most likely, the slant will be a new way of approaching an old problem.

2. Know your audience. The thrust of your presentation will differ enormously depending on who your target audience is. If you are writing for the general public, you will be doubly sure to refrain from technical jargon, and you will have to immediately catch your audience's attention and keep it throughout. The public can always change the station if they get the least bit bored, and they will. Although graduate or undergraduate students are a captive audience, they can still turn you off mentally and drift into thoughts of where they will be eating their dinner later. Graduate students require a different level of complexity than do undergraduates, who may be compared to a general audience. Continuing education for peers in your profession is probably the most common application of the teleclass, and you must be careful not to insult their current level of knowledge while providing them with relevant, new information.

3. Survey your audience. The expenditure of time and money for your project necessitates extreme care in the production of your project. You will want to be certain the interest or need is there before going ahead with production. Unless you are certain that your tape will feed a clearcut need, you should first survey the general needs in your field and produce a program to fill these needs. This is especially important if you wish to make your tape commercially available at some

time. Because budgets are usually low, an extensive written survey may not be feasible; a telephone survey of the prospective target populations may suffice. After the script is written, you may wish to have consultants and a sample of prospective viewers give feedback as to both accuracy and interest level. This may save expensive editing later.

4. Find a director and/or production company. There are production companies which specialize in creating films and videotapes for mental health purposes. Note programs you may have seen and find out who produced them. Talk to writers or producers and get information on how good a working relationship they had with the production company. The least expensive route is to find a director just starting out who wishes to add credits to his or her resume. These may be people who are connected with the industry through one of the more technical positions, often seen as stepping stones to more creative work. More likely you will find directors just starting out at local university film and television departments. If you choose one of these, be cautious; ask to see some things he or she has produced before. If you decide to go the amateur route, you may be able to find someone who will work for expenses only.

A second route is to hire a professional production company. This will be considerably more expensive, but you are also more likely to have a finer finished product.

If you are planning to show your production to a general audience, there is a third route available. This route is the commercial television stations and the cable networks. Because FCC regulations require a certain percentage of air time be devoted to public service, local stations occasionally produce their own public service messages. If your presentation falls under this category, you may be able to negotiate with a local station to produce your script for you. There are two important considerations. When assigned to a director under the employ of a commercial station, input into the program is highly dependent upon the idiosyncracies of the director, and it is likely that your input will be minimal. This route is also clouded by the hectic and capricious politics of commercial television, and anyone venturing into this realm should be prepared for anything.

Currently, the cable televison route is wide open. How long this trend will last is difficult to know, but there are at present many local cable television stations which will provide directors, and even equipment, for programs in which they are interested. One limitation to this route is the fact that the viewing audience can be highly restricted.

5. Construct a budget. A budget should be constructed in col-

laboration with the director. Only a professional director is familiar with the costs and the processes necessary to complete your presentation. In consultation with the director you will need to consider variables such as the ratio of location to studio shooting time, the kind of equipment necessary, the number of cameras, the kind and number of personnel required, props, uniforms, and coffee for actors, long-distance phone calls, and transportation costs.

6. Find the money. In these poor economic times, this is the most depressing task. Money can come from your own pocket, local, federal, or state grants, private foundations, commercial network support, or grants from the institution or department with which you are affiliated. As human service funding declines, these funds are drying up. A magical blend of luck, tenacity, creativity, savvy, and connections is required to fund such a venture. Good luck!

7. Choosing actors. If you are portraying some aspect of psychotherapy, you must decide whether to use actors or to use actual clients. Although clients' identities can be disguised through careful camera work, in my opinion it is not worth the effort to do so when actors can accomplish similar goals without the loss of information as valuable as facial expression. Actors are trained well in the portrayal of emotion, and they often surprise experienced therapists in their ability to capture the essence of the clients they portray. In this regard, I also believe that it is preferable not to work from scripts if at all possible. Actors should be given detailed descriptions of the roles they are to portray, as well as the situations they are in, and should be left to their own spontaneity in creating the role. This makes for a much more realistic portrayal of psychotherapy.

When actual clients are being used for demonstration purposes, extreme care must be taken to receive adequate informed consent. Consider the fact that clients are often well-behaved when placed in front of the video camera; the positive attention and the demand characteristics to appear healthy frequently contribute to frustrating, brief flights into health. Therefore, you may find yourself eventually looking for clients who give exaggerated performances in order to insure that you will end up with a satisfactory product.

8. Final edit. The final step to video production is the editing of the master videotape. In this aspect of producing your videotape, you may find your clinical sensitivities strained in an attempt to make the final product entertaining. Dull moments are best placed in the circular file, yet by doing so your final result loses realism for the sake of interest.

In the editing phase, the importance of good audio quality will become apparent. Audiotape recordings of videotape can be used for editing purposes, for it is easier to recall the sequence of events and maintain continuity with sound than it is with sight. Furthermore, inaudible moments tend to anger viewers more than does an occasional out-of-focus shot (Forrest et al., 1974).

If appropriate, the final tape can be transferred to film in order to serve as a master appropriate for making 16-mm films.


## Programmed Self-instruction

Programmed videotape instruction consists of a student viewing a videotape with specific learning goals and responding concurrently to a written instructional manual or checklist. The videotape may then give the student feedback, thus completing the input–practice–feedback cycle that is typical of programmed learning strategies.

Because programmed videotapes are expensive and time consuming to make, they are best suited to those subjects in which information does not change rapidly. Subjects that are highly dependent on observation—for example, the mental status interview—are also ideally suited for programmed videotapes.

An example of a series of self-instructional videotapes is that made by Suess (1973). The topics included sensorium, thought processes, mood and affect, and interpersonal relations. Each 45-minute video-tape began with a brief review of the information presented in the previous tape, followed by an explanation of the particular area of mental status under discussion at the time. This was presented along with the best examples of interviews taken from an extensive videotape library. The demonstration interview segments lasted from 30 to 90 seconds and were chosen to demonstrate a precise aspect of the mental status interview. As the students watched these short segments, they were encouraged to complete check-off sheets, designed to elicit certain student observations. Following each interview segment, the video monitor presented a picture of the same check-off sheet completed correctly. Each session ended with a review of what was taught in that videotape and a discussion of how the particular topic related to the overall process of psychodiagnostics. At the end of each class period, the instructor responded to any questions the students may have had about the videotape. (Notably, when the mental status course taught solely by videotape was compared with a control course taught with more traditional methods, achievement in both courses was the same. Those students who could not complete the regular course used the video self-instructional course as a make-up program.)

Suess noted seven advantages of self-instructional videotapes:

1. Because videotape can incorporate various other media, it offers a greater sensory range than do the printed word, the standard lecture, or audiotape self-instruction.
2. The low-cost availability of cassette recorders places self-instructional programs within the reach of most medical centers and clinics.
3. Programs that are planned and produced carefully can be used repeatedly, each time offering the same level of educational sophistication.
4. Videotapes are easily and quickly available to students who need to use them for purposes of make-up or studying.
5. They are available for later review by students.
6. A wide range of curricula is suited for programmed instruction.
7. Programmed instruction permits better utilization of teaching time by allowing the instructor to devote more time to individual student needs.

Suess also lists the following disadvantages:

1. Self-instructional videotapes are expensive to produce.
2. To assure a high-quality product, technical personnel and adequate videotaping equipment must be available.
3. No single source is likely to produce the wide variety of videotapes useful within a particular program. It is therefore important to make videotapes available within a distribution network. (See Appendix for sources of educational videotapes.)

Another model of programmed instruction was developed by Adler, Ware, and Enelow (1970). Their course in medical interviewing consisted of ten simulated interviews, each of which was designed to teach a single interviewing principle. Each videotaped interview gave the viewer the opportunity to select from among different interviewer reactions. After the student selected what he or she thought the interviewer should do at a particular point in the interview, two types of feedback were given on tape. First, the consequences of each choice were shown on the tape, and second, the instructor explained why one alternative was more effective than another.

## Videotape Libraries

Videotape libraries are valuable sources of clinical material for both training and treatment purposes. Videotapes can be obtained from three sources: They can be produced by the university, clinic, or hospital at which the library is located; they can be bought from commercial suppliers; or they can be on loan from other libraries or suppliers.

Commercially produced educational tapes, many of which are extremely valuable for teaching special topics, are available from a wide variety of sources. See Appendix for a list of some of these sources.

Videotape libraries can be used by students for the following purposes:

1. Case Material. There is often a serious lack of readily available clinical case material and suitable demonstrations of the type needed for a specific class. Videotapes can be made when case material is at hand and these can then be edited, coded, indexed, and stored for future use.

At a large university, both the psychiatric and psychological clinics see a large number of cases. Because of this, it is possible to develop a comprehensive permanent library that includes interviews with clients suffering from both basic and unusual disturbances. In order to do this, however, it is necessary that someone be responsible for screening clients for whether or not they are appropriate for videotaping.

These videotapes can be used to supplement the education of clinicians who might otherwise have access to only a limited number of clients. For example, students doing internships at small, regional hospitals may find themselves lacking in experience with certain populations. These students can use the videotape library of a large university hospital to learn the symptomatology of cases with which the student is unfamiliar. Or else the local clinic may be the recipient of an interlibrary loan, enabling the student to view the videotapes at the regional clinic. Videotape is also especially useful in instances of acute disturbance. Because the flare-up is so infrequent, it is likely that an intern may not have the opportunity to experience such an episode.

2. Extra credit. Advanced students may consult videotaped material in specialized topics to receive extra credit in undergraduate classes.

3. Test administration. Tapes demonstrating the administration of various psychological tests can be enormously helpful as an adjunct to courses in assessment. This is especially true in the case of infrequently used or highly specialized test materials which the instructor may not wish to take the time to demonstrate.

4. Make-up. Students who miss class lectures can watch videotapes of those lectures for make-up purposes.

5. Special lectures. Seminars and lectures given by visiting professors can be taped and kept for students who could not be at the original class or lecture. When particular tapes are found to be highly valuable, they can be incorporated into the curriculum of the relevant course.

6. The long view. Every library designed for use in training psychotherapists should have, at the very least, one set of tapes which, taken together, represent a client's progress over time. This, of course, permits students to get a sense of the long-term process of psychotherapy. Ideally, a good videotape library should have several of these sets available for student use, including different diagnostic categories and different treatment modalities.

Typically, videotape libraries have been concerned with providing material for students, interns, residents, and trainees who might benefit from them. Lately, however, there is increasing opportunities for utilization of libraries directly by clients. Treatment settings should consider the following direct uses of video libraries by clients:

1. Relaxation training. A client could be assigned a specific tape or set of tapes instructing the client in methods of relaxation.

2. Vicarious desensitization. Videotaped desensitization hierarchies (Chapter 2, p. 18) could be provided on loan to those clients who wish to practice at home.

3. Client education. Clients who suffer from particular disorders can frequently benefit from videotapes that teach the client about that disorder. One example mentioned is the use of tapes in dealing with certain aspects of sexual dysfunction (see Chapter 8, p. 165). Parents of children with such problems as enuresis or Tourette's syndrome may also benefit from learning about these problems through videotapes.

The chief drawback of the videotape library is its expense. Videotape costs have remained fairly stable over the last few years and are currently much less expensive than they were only a decade ago. Nevertheless, a videotape library involves a collection of a large number of tapes which, taken together, represent a considerable investment. One possible solution, although time-consuming, is to make a concerted effort to edit only those portions of therapy sessions useful for training purposes and to then condense these into fewer tapes.

A second and related disadvantage is that videotape libraries tie up videotapes which could potentially be reused repeatedly for other purposes. It may be wiser to arrange a mutual borrowing system if you are located near a large medical center or university facility that may already have a well-stocked library.

## Simulation

Generally stated, video simulation is the combination of roleplaying and videotape; when added to lectures and class discussion it is a very powerful means of learning practical skills (Froelich, 1978; Froelich & Bishop, 1969; Ramey, 1968). First the teacher must choose a situation likely to be encountered by the student. This situation should engender role conflict with no clearcut, appropriate response pattern. The teacher then sets the stage, defining the time and place of the situation as well as the roles of the people involved in coping with the problem at hand. The roleplayers are selected from the class, and each is given identical, brief statements of the problem. In Ramey's version, roleplayers are given a written case outline with enough advance notice to study it, as well as related readings.

Each role player is then given a sealed envelope that contains a one-paragraph description further defining his or her feelings, attitudes, and position regarding the problem. If warranted, roleplayers are given any further information that they might have access to in real life (for example, lab reports, diagnoses, or demographic data). The role player is then free to develop the role as he or she wishes. Ramey uses a standard second paragraph indicating that the role is open-ended and that the role player is instructed to draw on experience, training, and development of the situation. The role players are discouraged from discussing the problem at hand prior to videotaping the first inter-action.

The teacher functions primarily as a director. At first the instructor calls into the room only those players who are in the first scene. Other players are separated in order to avoid the embarrassment of performing before uninvolved peers and to prevent others who may be involved from knowing what occurs prior to their entrance onto the scene. Other than chairs, props are usually not needed.

When the scene has come to a natural endpoint, the instructor calls a halt. Otherwise a role player may request permission to see another role player who may be waiting in an adjacent room with the others who are not involved in the current scene. The videotape is then begun and scene two is recorded when the appropriate players are available.

The lengths of individual scenes vary, as does the number of scenes required to complete a simulation. A completed simulation may run anywhere from 10 minutes to an hour, although Froelich's simulations typically run between 20 and 30 minutes.

There should be a delay between completion of the simulation and replay before the class of at least 12 hours. This gives role players time to detach themselves from their roles and to rest before class. The added sense of detachment gives those who participate an increased feeling of freedom to express both positive and negative feelings about the simulation.

Prior to or at the outset of class, students are given copies of the original statement of the problem, and they are asked to discuss the difficulties they think might arise and how they think the role players will act. After this overview the videotaped simulation is replayed for the entire class, with all members of the class given permission to interrupt or stop the tape at any time to make a comment or ask a question.

The artful execution of this discussion, occurring before, during, and after the replay of the video simulation, is the core of the learning process. The professor must facilitate discussion, raise important points, encourage insights, listen, and manipulate the tape recorder.

The class should have between an hour and a half to three hours to work through a complete video simulation. A brief example, quoted in part from Ramey (1968), might help to visualize this particular activity:

> In this small community hospital setting many physicians seem to follow the local cultural norm of avoiding any talk of death until the last possible moment, but others say that the patient should always be told he is dying as soon as the doctor is reasonably sure.
>
> The new attending has gotten himself in a bit of a bind with his first terminal patient. He is not convinced that it is to the patient's benefit to tell him he is probably not going to leave the hospital alive. The patient's wife appears to believe that telling him such a thing would "put the black hand on him." But the nurse on the case appears to be surprised that the patient has not been told. The father of the patient has been urging the doctor to inform his son regarding the true nature of his illness for over a week. At what point should the decision be made? The doctor is in a quandary. (p. 57)

The roles that are assigned include that of the young physician, an experienced nurse, a wife afraid that the truth might hurt her husband's recovery, and the father. The nurse and physician are told that the intent of the first take is to provide an opportunity to set the stage and articulate their positions in global terms. This process is open-ended and takes only a few minutes.

In the second take, the nurse talks briefly to the patient prior to the doctor entering the scene and then stands by as the physician talks to the patient. The physician, in this example, chose not to disclose that the patient was terminally ill. The patient nevertheless attempted to get the physician to tell him about his illness.

The nurse was confronted by the patient's wife and parents in the third take. The wife and parents had extreme difficulty facing the fact that the patient was on his deathbed. The doctor soon arrived and appeared bewildered by the family's insistence on avoiding the topic of death. The wife finally accused the physician of treating the patient like an animal. The physician turned away, and remarked, "We're not treating him like an animal." He then turned toward the wife and said, "If he were an animal, we would put him out of his misery!"

On playback, the class discussed the ramifications of the physician's remarks. An attempt was made to relate theoretical considerations to practical implications and to have this occur in a situation in which students could experience the feelings involved in roleplays.

One of the essential tenets of video simulation is the notion that the most effective learning occurs in situations that are similar to those in which the information is expected to be used. Furthermore, video simulation is best accomplished when the following steps are adhered to in proper sequence: the performance of the skill; accurate feedback; a change in the second performance; and feedback on the second performance. Without this double practice it is likely that a student will repeatedly continue to make the same mistakes.

## Stimulus-response Tapes

The use of stimulus-modeling tapes in group therapy was discussed earlier in Chapter 4. Stimulus tape techniques provide some of the finest training experiences available to students; they give students the opportunity to react to a clinical situation without the fear of making costly mistakes.

Stimulus tapes are short, videotaped vignettes that portray significant situations that the therapist might encounter. They are excellent means of exploring underlying attitudes and values, the clarification of which plays a central part in the training of a mental health professional. Stimulus tapes are most often made from the "subjective camera" viewpoint in which the actor speaks directly into the camera as if relating directly to the viewer. Sometimes a large video screen is used to enhance realism. Following the brief vignette, the trainee or class is called upon to respond in one of the following ways:

1. Class members are asked to think about, and perhaps write, what they should say or do next. It is important to elicit how students felt as they listened to the stimulus tape, especially since many tapes may tap into countertransference conflicts. The instructor may then compare the responses within a class discussion.

2. After the vignette is shown, a videotape is made of the trainee responding to the vignette. For example, if the stimulus tape concerns a client posing a question, the student–therapist responds immediately following presentation of the vignette. A videotape made of this response could then be replayed either to the student alone or to a group of students who comment upon the implications and motivations of the response.

3. A group is divided into pairs, and each partner is labeled either number one or two. Following presentation of the stimulus tape, partner number one continues in the client role as depicted in the brief vignette. Partner number two responds as he or she would in the role of the therapist. Following this roleplay, each dyad discusses the process, explores each member's feelings, and discusses alternatives. The instructor may wish to have dyad members discuss their effective and ineffective strategies with the whole group, and perhaps provide an opportunity to roleplay once more, practicing more effective strategies.

Following is a list of some suggested stimulus tape vignettes:

1. An adolescent boy looks at you angrily and says: "Okay. So I stole the money from my teacher. She'll never know, and you better not ever tell her. Besides, she's a creep and she deserves it. But if my mother ever finds out, my dad will kill me. I know you talk to my dad about stuff, are you gonna tell him I stole the three hundred dollars?"

2. A middle-aged man looks at you calmly and incredulously. He says, "You're not Jewish, are you? I hope not, because I hate Jews. All of them. Some people think I'm a bigot, but I don't! I think they *all* should have been killed. When you think they all should have been killed, you're not prejudiced! (He laughs.)

3. A woman in her mid-twenties begins to sob. "This is our first session, and I'm not sure I trust you. I've never told this to anyone before, but when I was thirteen, my father raped me. Ever since then

I've felt worthless and empty inside. And I can't trust anyone. All my relationships with men have been a disaster."

4. "Suicide? Sure, I've thought about suicide often. Every night. Every day. There isn't a day that goes by that I haven't thought of jumping out of my window at work, or stepping out in front of a car."

5. "Michael said you told him he didn't need to be in therapy. Is that true? If he doesn't need to be in therapy, then you must be ripping us off."

6. A young man looks at you with a sad, pleading expression on his face. He quietly and sincerely says, "I've been seeing you now for over a year and a half. This is very hard for me, but I have something I have to tell you. I don't know what you'll think of me. I've been having these dreams ever since I started seeing you. I dream that you're torturing me. But then we make love. I'm very confused."

7. "I overheard you talking about me in the coffeeshop. I'm furious! That's against the law, it must be, but that's not the worst part. The worst part is that you were making fun of me. You mentioned my name, I heard it, and you were laughing about me. I don't know what to do. I know I have to stop therapy . . . I'm too mad at you to go on. But I don't know if I should sue you or not. I really feel like it, but I have to talk to a lawyer and find out if it's feasible."

Vignettes may be prepared that respond specifically to the needs of a class. For example, vignette 7 above is appropriate for a class in ethical issues. A stock of vignettes may be used for general courses in psychotherapy, courses in crisis intervention, or in training in specific theoretical approaches. In the latter case, stimulus tapes are excellent vehicles for exploring the relationship between theory and practice.

As with video simulations, the stimulus tape is produced using a subjective camera point of view and makes liberal use of close-ups revealing affect laden facial expression. Fadeouts may be used at the end of each tape to cue the viewer that the vignette is ending and that a response is called for.

## The Video Examination

Evaluation of students in the clinical area is a difficult procedure; traditional paper and pencil tests can tap the quantity of knowledge retained but do little to assess one's ability to apply that knowledge to actual clinical problems.

The ideal clinical examination would entail a student actually interviewing a client under unobtrusive faculty observation. While this can be accomplished with videotape methods, there are two serious drawbacks; it is often difficult or impossible to find suitable clients at the time and place (and in the numbers) they are needed for exam purposes, and the use of different clients does not permit standardized testing procedures.

The videotest was designed to ameliorate these difficulties. The version designed by Weir (1975, 1978), along with alternative strategies, is discussed below.

Weir's test consists of three five-minute videotaped segments of previously recorded patient interviews. When combined with a written examination instrument, the examination provides a test of the student's ability to apply knowledge obtained in the course to the observation of a client presenting a clinical problem.

The test can be administered either individually or in groups. Each five-minute segment is played for the students and then stopped. They are then given 20 minutes to do a writeup on the patient, including responses to the following questions:

1. List behavioral and mental status features demonstrated by the patient. Include positive and negative features, as appropriate, using proper terminology.
2. Differential diagnosis. Given the behavioral and mental status material noted above, make a differential diagnosis using proper terminology. Be as specific as possible. Circle the single most likely diagnosis in your opinion.
3. Case management. Write a brief paragraph. Discuss what type of therapy might be indicated on the basis of your primary diagnostic impression. Be specific; if drugs are prescribed, what drug and in what dosage? If psychotherapy, what type? Should the patient be hospitalized; for what reason? Are further studies indicated; if so, what studies and for what purpose? Be brief and specific.

The examinees are shown the first patient only once in an attempt to assess the acuteness of the students' perceptions. After 20 minutes, the same procedure is followed with the last two segments. The entire examination takes about one and a quarter hours to complete. Because students have great interest in reviewing the material after the examination period, the professor should leave 15 to 30 minutes to review the videotape and discuss the diagnostic and observational process.

One of the main considerations in the preparation of a videotest is the selection of the test material. It is important that the instructor clearly define the level of acumen expected of the student, and that he or she then structure the test so that it is commensurate with these expectations. Another consideration is the length of the segments to be used. A long segment may be used to test the depth of knowledge with a certain type of client or a certain problem, or short, edited segments may be used to test a wider breadth of knowledge within a certain global field. Brief segments typically can be edited from longer segments in ways that preserve the integrity of the processes being examined.

Good technical quality is important in order to allow the student to take advantage of such subtle cues as vocal intonation and small motor movements. Contradictory material should be avoided as well, in order to increase both the heuristic value and the validity of the test.

Special techniques—fades, pan shots, and split-screens—should be avoided because they alter the clinical realism of the presentation. Furthermore, changes in camera angle or distance (close-up versus long shots) should be minimal; this gives the observer the choice of focusing on aspects of the image that he or she deems important.

Content validity of the material should be ascertained by showing the videotaped segments to several faculty members. Agreement as to scope and relevance of the material should be high. Furthermore, the faculty members could be given the test themselves; differences among them could be used as a basis for clarifying test questions, re-editing, or replacing videotaped segments. Faculty responses to questions could also be used as a scoring profile for the students. Suess (1973), for example, gave his version of a videotest to his department's senior staff in psychiatry and psychology. Only those items which received 85 percent or better staff agreement were used as the solution for student grading purposes.

Another way of constructing videotests is to combine the observation of interviews with standardized rating instruments of psychopathology. For example, Tardiff (1981) has used both the Global Adaptation Scale (GAS) and the Lorr Inpatient Multidimensional Psychiatric Scale (IMPS) to measure medical students' abilities to observe psychopathology. Students' ratings on the IMPS, for example, are compared with combined independent ratings made by the students' supervisors. Any item that does not elicit at least 80 percent agreement among the supervisors is eliminated.

## Big Brother

The use of closed-circuit television as a "spying" device is a somewhat controversial issue. It is reminiscent of Orwell's "big brother," and it conjures up questions of invasion of privacy. Privacy is a right patients in a mental hospital deserve, but there are times when absolute privacy puts the patient at greater risk than he or she ought to be.

One of the best uses of video in a hospital facility is in its isolation or "seclusion" rooms. All mental hospitals have them; they are the places patients who are imminently dangerous to themselves or others are placed to keep them away from their fellow patients and under the watchful eye of the staff. Unfortunately, however, patients in seclusion are often forgotten or are left unobserved for longer periods of time than they should be.

A video camera located in a seclusion room could be linked to a monitor in the nurse's station where the patient could be observed continuously, or with a mere glance upwards from a chart.

While I was working as a psychology intern in a large state mental hospital in California, a patient with whom I had been closely working died. He died while in seclusion, and to this day the cause of his death remains a mystery. One thing remains clear, however; had he been observed he probably would have not died so soon before his time. At the time of his death the ward was bustling. It was shift turnover and new patients were being admitted. John was in isolation for multiple suicide threats and various attempts; although the law required that he be checked every fifteen minutes, John had spent so much time in seclusion he was merely forgotten. The next time he was observed he was seen aspirating. By that time efforts to revive him were fruitless.

Providing a monitor in a nurse's station does not assure that it will be watched. The chances of patients going unobserved for a long period of time, however, would be reduced. Unusual patient behavior would probably catch the eye of a passing observer.

# 8

# Special Populations

Up to this point the activities in this book have been categorized by the general therapeutic modalities for which they are appropriate. Where a particular activity is more germane for highly regressed individuals than "normal neurotics" or for a certain age group, this has been specified. Other than these general categories, specific client populations have not been isolated. This chapter discusses the use of video with specific target populations—groups of people whose symptoms often require specialized treatment methods. It is well known that certain psychotherapeutic orientations and interventions are more effective with some presenting problems than with others. For example, clients with discrete phobias are more likely to respond favorably to counterconditioning therapies than to insight-oriented psychodynamic therapies. For the alcoholic, it is necessary to strongly confront the stubborn denial mechanisms employed to shield the alcoholic from his or her intense fear and rage. The effects of the alcoholic's behavior while intoxicated are easy to deny, for they are often lost to amnesia when the alcoholic is sober. The sober alcoholic's viewing of his or her drunken comportment can go further in defeating denial than can a therapist's insistent verbal prods. Similarly, the sufferer of seizure disorders often forgets the premonitory signs; video replays can help this person learn what environmental and emotional cues may prompt a seizure so that those cues may be avoided in the future.

Other groups require other special treatment methods. This chapter discusses some suggested uses of video in the treatment of alcoholism, seizure disorders, anorexia nervosa, and Tourette's syndrome. Also discussed are some ways of incorporating video feedback in assertion training groups, parent training, and sex therapy, as well as a novel way of incorporating video feedback into the inpatient treatment of a person who has recently attempted suicide. This is meant to be only a sample of the specific problems with which video can be used. Some of the more rare disorders—multiple personality, for example—have also responded to video feedback (cf. Berger, 1978), but because of their low incidence these will not be discussed in detail here.

There are, to my knowledge, few populations which will not in some way respond to video feedback. As mentioned earlier, video should be used cautiously with suicidal individuals who may use the video feedback to confirm their self-hatred, and with those who are in an acute psychotic state. Even with these individuals, however, video may be used fruitfully; for the depressed, suicidal individual video can help the therapist in directly confronting the irrational beliefs underlying faulty self-perceptions, and for the psychotic individual video can be used to confront the client with his or her bizarre and maladaptive defenses when he or she is in a more lucid, receptive state.

In all of the special populations mentioned above, video is used as a tool along with other specialized techniques, most often in combination with behavioral interventions and/or insight-oriented verbal psychotherapy. At the risk of being repetitive, it is important that video be considered only one step in the comprehensive treatment programs that are often required to alleviate some of the severe problems discussed in this chapter.

# The Populations

## The Suicidal Patient

As an example of how video can be used with suicidal patients, Resnik, Davison, Schuyler, and Christopher (1973) described their use of video with patients brought into the emergency room of the National Naval Medical Center in Bethesda, Maryland. When a patient arrives after attempting suicide, an on-call videotape team is alerted. The team obtains consent from either the patient (if possible) or a relative. A videotape is then made of the patient's condition on arrival, the complete procedures used to save his or her life, interactions with hospital personnel, and the reactions of family and friends. An emphasis is made on close-up shots of both the patient's and the family's facial expressions.

When patients are capable, they are transferred to the hospital's psychiatry service where they receive group and individual psychotherapy. After two individual psychotherapy sessions, the patient is brought to a quiet viewing room with subdued lighting. There, patients are shown a ten-minute segment of the emergency room videotape. (Measurements are also made of the patient's galvanic skin response, and given the "state" scale of the State–Trait Anxiety Inventory in order to gauge the patient's anxiety level during the viewing of the videotape.) Thereafter, the patient is brought back to view the videotape of the emergency room procedures following every two individual psychotherapy sessions. This pattern continues until the patient's anxiety decreases significantly in the judgment of the treatment team and as measured by skin response. The authors argue that the patient's ability to see him or herself undergo such procedures as tracheotomies, gastric lavage, receiving oxygen, and being sutured aids in confronting the denial of suicide intent and despair by demonstrating the consequences of his or her behavior. This serves to motivate patients into accepting responsibility for the self-destructive aspects of their personality and their ambivalence about living. This responsibility for self-destructiveness decreases resistance to the therapeutic process; therefore, patients who receive video feedback typically engage in a therapeutic alliance sooner than do other suicide attempters and are more apt to give up their unproductive defenses. In fact, they notice that often the exposure to the emergency room tape brings relevant material to the surface that helps engage patients in a therapeutic alliance.

A frequent response to the initial videotape exposure is one of hostility toward the therapist. Patients may feel tricked by the therapist or may transfer their fears, guilt, and shame into anger. This hostility is typically manageable in therapy and tends to stimulate salient interpretations and insights valuable in the patients' psychotherapeutic work.

Videotape self-confrontation is only a first step. Each confrontation must be seen within the context of the psychotherapy session and the overall treatment program. A supportive therapeutic network is required to deal with the intense self-hatred and underlying conflicts that are likely to be uncovered in the videotape confrontation process.

There are a variety of patients who may benefit from this type of emergency room confrontation. Included may be the juvenile diabetic or the epileptic who is recurrently brought into the emergency room in coma. These patients may be confronted with the results of failure to take their medication in a way that they may be unable to experience otherwise.

## Seizure Disorders

This four-stage technique was developed by Feldman and Paul (1976) in order to reduce the frequency of seizures in epileptic patients. It is particularly appropriate for those epileptics in whom psychogenic factors are strong influences in the onset of seizures.

The first phase is the exploratory phase which consists of interviewing the patient in order to confirm the neurological background and to obtain a case history of recurrent seizures. The main thrust of this phase (which is not videotaped) is to recognize a pattern of association between the occurrence of seizures and stressful environmental stimuli. The environmental stimuli may include particular stressful situations and/or specific interpersonal relationships. Such variables as frequency of occurrence, duration, prior treatment, age of onset, and clinical manifestations are investigated. Corroborative evidence from family members and previous physicians, as well as electroencephalographic evidence are also obtained during this phase. Of special importance is inquiry into the occurrence of seizures and their timing in relationship to environmental circumstances that may be of special significance to the patient.

The second phase is the stimulated recall phase. During this stage videotape or audiotape recordings of conversations of unidentified people which stimulate various intensities of emotional responses are presented to both the patient and the patient's family members. For example, if it is determined during the exploratory phase that the patient has an emotional vulnerability regarding mother–daughter relationships, a tape may be played of a mother and daughter, of ages similar to the patient and the patient's mother (or daughter), in which the two discuss the overprotectiveness of the mother toward the daughter. These recordings are called stressor tapes. They contain selected emotional sets directed toward eliciting particular feelings and toward stimulating the patient to recall a previously unexperienced emotion. Various stressor tapes are selected and presented in a systematic fashion based on the data obtained during the exploratory phase. This process may occur over a period of several sessions. The purpose of presenting this material is to stimulate or precipitate a clinical seizure. When a seizure is in fact precipitated by a particular tape, this tape is used again in later sessions for confirming the effects of stimulated recall. The facial expression and verbalizations of the patient while watching the stressor tapes are videotaped for later review by the patient.

The third phase is the self-confrontation phase, and it too occurs over a period of several visits. During this stage the videotape of the patient reacting to the effective stressor tape is shown to the patient. The central point of this self-confrontation is to provide the patient with a glimpse of the experiences and responses that are typically lost to epileptics due to ictal amnesia. The reactions the patient has to viewing the videotape of the seizure are also recorded. This recording is then shown to the patient using a split-screen format (see Chapter 9) with one half showing the intentionally provoked seizure and the other half showing the patient watching the seizure. Again, the responses of the patient are recorded, and the events observed during each interview are discussed with the patient. (These discussions typically reveal a heightened awareness of the actual circumstances that triggered the seizure.)

The fourth phase is called the reminding phase. During the self-confrontation phase, an association is made by the patient between the specific emotional trigger and the events precipitating the seizure. This knowledge is periodically reinforced during the reminding phase in order to alert the patient to the presence of his or her emotional triggers. The client reviews the split-screen recording of the seizure along with the patient's reaction to it or else simply listens to the audio recording of the interviews. This process reinforces the insight acquired during the previous phases of the technique. In time, the patient's awareness of the kinds of situations or interpersonal relationships capable of precipitating a seizure permits the patient to avoid responding in the same emotional way that typically provokes seizures.

The originators of this technique report significantly reduced seizure activity among those with whom it has been attempted. It is a potentially powerful tool which may permit patients to deal with issues provoked by the video replay that may not have been available to them in attempts at psychotherapy due to both the ictal and retrograde amnesia resulting from the epilepsy. The therapeutic value of the video self-confrontation process seems to result from the ability to actually see oneself responding during exposure to stressful antecedent stimuli, and the ability to associate the emotionally upsetting antecedents with the onset of a seizure. This permits patients to either consciously avoid the kinds of events that may be potentially harmful to them or to muster alternative ways of coping with the stress.

## Video Techniques with Alcoholics

The world of the alcoholic is filled with denial, self-hatred, tenaciously unfulfilled dependency needs, and fears of meeting those needs with intimacy. Videotape techniques in which the alcoholic is confronted with his or her intoxicated behavior have been an important facet in the treatment of alcoholism for many clinicians. The applicability of this approach is due largely to the necessity of breaking down the alcoholic's extremely stubborn denial system.

Among alcoholics there tends to be a large discrepancy between self-perception and the way the alcoholic is perceived by others. There is also a discrepancy between outward expression of feeling and the internal experience of feelings. The alcoholic is one who may appear self-confident while concealing tremendous insecurity and dependency needs, or may appear happy while concealing depression. Confronting an alcoholic with his or her self-image helps to bring these conflicts to a sober awareness that is often blurred in inebriation. Confronting an alcoholic with his or her self-image also gives the client the opportunity to build a conscious bridge between the "sober self" and the intoxicated self that is frequently lost to alcoholic amnesia.

It has been demonstrated in many of the studies utilizing video self-confrontation techniques with alcoholics that the experience often helps them to more readily accept subsequent psychotherapy. Furthermore, several users of this technique report another curious advantage; interviewing a client while intoxicated often facilitates the emergence of psychodynamically relevant information which would be more difficult to ascertain within the constraints of sobriety.

As with many of the other populations with which video is used, the most effective treatment for alcoholism is a comprehensive one. Video confrontation can be considered only a facet of the treatment of alcoholism, one which may function best as an initial component in the alcoholic's treatment program.

There has been a wide variety of videotape applications to the treatment of alcoholism. Each, in some way, revolves around confronting the alcoholic with his or her behavior while intoxicated, either mildly so (see for example, Paredes, Ludwig, Hassenfeld, & Cornelison, 1969) or extremely so (for example, Feinstein & Tamerin, 1972; Vogler & Caddy, 1973).

A well-designed study, incorporating video feedback as an initial treatment component, was conducted by Baker, Udin, and Vogler (1975) at Patton State Hospital in California. This study found that video self-confrontation combined with behavioral counseling was a more effective treatment strategy than was behavioral counseling alone, role-modeling, or standard inpatient treatment. Subjects receiving video feedback of their drinking behavior took more time to consume drinks than did any of the other subjects, consumed significantly fewer drinks than did the subjects who experienced a modeling treatment, and significantly increased the amount of sips they took to completely consume a drink. The videotape group also made more volitional follow-up contacts than did any of the other groups. The authors concluded that "videotape self-confrontation of drunken comportment should be an ideal initial component in a treatment program where subjects are provided with explicit behavioral goals and techniques" (p. 790). Other studies (for example, Vogler, Weissbach, & Compton, 1977) also demonstrate the relative superiority of video techniques in the treatment of alcoholics.

An initial consideration is where the first drinking sessions will occur. It is most informative to attempt, if possible, to simulate the environment in which the alcoholic has the most difficulty refraining from drinking. If most of the drinking occurs at home, it would be best to attempt to simulate a home environment. Family members, who may be involved in the treatment program, may borrow video equipment and tape the client while intoxicated at home. This, of course, requires the cooperation of the family, as well as the client, and the home environment must be amenable to this. If most of the abuse occurs in a bar, a simulated bar may be created in the treatment setting. If treatment is occurring in an alcohol detoxification unit, a client may be videotaped during the initial interview, in which case he or she may be intoxicated at the time, obviating the necessity to "get the client drunk."

Various studies utilized various kinds and amounts of alcohol. Some chose to serve only one drink of fixed alcoholic content repeatedly, in order to better compare reactions to the amount of alcohol consumed. For treatment purposes alone, this would be an unnecessary consideration. The most useful technique would be to encourage the client to imbibe as much as he or she wishes until intoxicated.

It may be a worthwhile step to videotape the client for a period of time prior to intoxication in order to compare this with the later, intoxicated state. After initial signs of intoxication, the videotape recorder is left running, and a taped record is made of the client's behavior while intoxicated. During this time, the therapist or interviewer may be obtaining general background information, or information that may shed light on the client's psychodynamics. This may help the therapist during playback, when the therapist may wish to compare the information given by the client while inebriated with the client's feelings about the information while sober. In such a context, recognition of distortions and deceptions may lead to important insights during playback.

Clients then view their drunken behavior immediately prior to counseling sessions. These sessions may include counseling in specific methods of generating alternate responses to stressors, delineating the reinforcers and consequences of inebriated behavior, and acquiring appropriate, controlled drinking patterns. It has been found to be helpful to include training in how to lengthen the time it takes to consume a drink (since most alcoholics are guzzlers), and increasing the number of sips required to consume a drink. Instruction on the minimum number of sips it takes to consume a drink, the kinds of drinks to order, proper dilution of drinks, and sensible cut-off points can also be provided (Sobell & Sobell, 1973). Written and experiential tests may also be used as a way of assuring that this information is learned (Baker et al., 1975), although this does not assure generalization of knowledge.

Feinstein and Tamerin (1972) presented a more psychodynamically oriented approach. They experimentally intoxicated a client for ten sessions over a five-week period. Sessions lasted an hour and a half two times a week. Following intoxication, the therapist conducted an individual psychotherapy session using the same techniques as were used previously with the client while sober. Instead of immediate feedback, the therapist reviewed the videotape recording for a two-hour period with the client on alternate days. In this particular single case study, the authors reported dramatic improvement during the five-week treatment period. Amnesia decreased, and the client became more insightful of his conflicts. He was more open, relaxed, and communicative when dealing with hospital staff and other patients. This improvement, however, was short-lived; the patient returned to his alcoholic behavior following discharge from the hospital.

An alternate approach is to videotape a client while intoxicated at admission to the hospital, then to replay the videotape to the client within a group therapy context (Faia & Shean, 1976). This permits the therapeutic aspects of video self-confrontation to be combined with the therapeutic aspects of group therapy—a support system, an opportunity to share experiences, feelings, and insights with others who have similar problems. Viewing videotapes within a group context can also help to enhance rapport among group members.

Viewing a videotape recording of intoxicated behavior in the presence of family members may also serve to increase the motivation of alcoholics to change, as well as providing a valuable, validating experience for the members of the family.

Because of the difficulties inherent in using alcohol as part of a treatment strategy, several cautions are advised. First, it is extremely important that clients receive a medical screening prior to a "therapeutic" drinking session. Second, in the event that a client becomes violent towards him- or herself or others, adequate staff should be available for handling such a crisis. Third, each client should be observed following a drinking session to be sure he or she does not leave the treatment setting while still intoxicated.

In one study (Schaefer, Sobell, & Mills, 1971) it was noted that self-confrontation actually accentuated post-treatment drinking, perhaps due to the stress it may have induced. The apparent reason for this, however, was the failure to intervene therapeutically on an ongoing basis following treatment. It is suggested that the most effective strategy would be to combine initial treatment with behavioral counseling and ongoing post-treatment follow-up of behavioral suggestions.

In the event that it is not feasible to undergo intoxication procedures such as those mentioned above, the use of a vicarious videotape technique may be substituted (see Chapter 2, p. 18). Otherwise, there is a simple, alternative way of using videotape in the treatment of alcoholics. As with most simple alternatives, it is probably not as effective as the more elaborate intoxication procedures. This alternative is to simply use modeling procedures, as did Greer and Callis (1975). They interviewed graduates of the Alcohol Treatment Program at the North Little Rock Veterans Administration Hospital and then showed these videotapes to the current treatment group over a 12-session period. In their interviews, graduates related what they did and didn't do in the program that contributed to successful discharge. They were then verbally reinforced whenever they mentioned a positive step they took. Following the presentation of each videotape, the current treatment group discussed their reactions to watching the tape. During this period, members of the treatment group were also reinforced for making references to any intention to behave in productive ways, that is, similar to the graduate model.

An incidental improvement in some of the clients with whom video feedback has been used was a reduction in obesity (Paredes, Gottheil, Tausig, & Cornelison, 1969). Confrontation with one's physical image can be a strong motivator for change in an area in which some clients may feel more in control. Others found that self-confrontation led to an increased awareness of expressive behavior that linked them with significant others, while others found in their reflected image the depth of their self-esteem. Most important, many alcoholics see in their self-image a source of insight into their conflicts and a stimulus for change.

## Anorexia Nervosa

She was extremely emaciated and so weak she could barely walk. Looking like a starved inmate of a concentration camp, she was nevertheless fearful lest she be made to eat and become fat. Her concern and her view of herself were clearly discrepant from the concerns and views of her family and physicians. Seeing herself daily in the mirror did not change her view of herself as being in danger of becoming obese. (Gottheil, Backup, & Cornelison, 1969, p. 238)

Such is the description of a 17-year-old anorexic woman at the beginning of her treatment with a unique form of "self-image confrontation." It consisted of conducting two types of standard sessions; the first was a behavioral recording (BR) session, in which the woman was asked the same questions: "How are you feeling today?" "How did you sleep last night?" "What time did you go to sleep?" "What time did you get up?" "When did you have your last meal?" "What did you have to eat?" "How did it taste?" "Would you please describe what you see in this room?"

These meetings were filmed with sound movie equipment. In the second session called the self-image experience (SIE) the patient was shown the film of her previous session, and she was asked the following contrived questions: "Who was the person in the picture?" "What was the person doing in the picture?" "What did you think of it?" "What did you like about the picture?" "What did you dislike about it?" "What would you like to change in it?" These sessions were also filmed.

The rationale for the contrived questions was to prevent a relationship from forming with the therapist who conducted these sessions, in order to not interfere with the concurrent psychotherapy which was conducted by a different therapist at a different institution. This was done in order to better evaluate the impact of the procedure on therapy, and vice versa.

After answering the questions, only trivial matters were discussed by the two, again in an effort to avoid the formation of a close relationship. An attempt was made, however, to create a congenial, accepting atmosphere.

The behavior recording sessions were conducted every other week, while the self-image confrontation was conducted weekly. On weeks in which both sessions occurred, the behavior recording preceded the feedback session. In the self-image confrontation, sometimes only a part of a behavior recording session would be replayed, while at other times the whole session would be replayed. After the fourteenth week, earlier films were alternated with more current ones in order to see the different responses the patient had to the same film segments at different stages in her treatment. Also, it was noted that the patient enjoyed seeing older films alternated with more recent ones because she could see the difference in her appearance and behavior over time. The complete treatment lasted for over a year.

Although the awkward, contrived format of the recording sessions proved to be repetitious, boring, and unresponsive to the immediate concerns of the patient, they did not interfere with the forming of a relationship between the patient and the interviewer. The questioning became a sort of ritual, which she could interrupt at any moment and return to later. The standard format was successful in providing a boundary between the interviewer and the client, for the interviewer could always return to the video replay when the patient began to discuss issues that might compete with the psychotherapeutic relationship.

At the outset of the self-image confrontation, the patient was able to completely deny that she saw anything that disturbed her about her emaciated appearance. After repeated confrontations, however, her satisfaction with her self-image turned to disinterest and boredom. She then became hostile toward the procedure and rejected her image. Nevertheless, she willingly continued to participate in the filming procedure. Later in the course of treatment the patient became better able to take an objective stance toward her image. This coincided with an increased ability to attend to aspects of her personality other than her weight. She began to experiment with the camera, finding new ways to express herself and trying these out. Interestingly, when the patient became able to see both positive and negative aspects of herself in the self-image confrontation, she also began to express positive and negative feelings toward her parents in the individual therapy session.

Through repeated self-confrontation, the patient learned that when she was emaciated she looked pathetic. She also learned that when she was disturbed about her self-image, she could not see the relation between being thin and not eating. Toward the end of her treatment, however, she was amazed to see how she could have viewed herself looking so emaciated at the beginning and not be disturbed.

Several factors seemed less than ideal in the implementation of this treatment strategy. Because the authors used film instead of video, one day to one week was required for processing the film before the image could be seen by the patient. It is possible that either immediate self-confrontation or videotaped replays could have substantially shortened the length of time it took to make progress.

Furthermore, the research emphasis and probably the theoretical orientation of the authors led to what I think was an overconcern with compromising the primary psychotherapeutic relationship. If the video feedback was conducted by the primary therapist, the link between the client's appearance and the issues being discussed could have been stronger. This, combined with the immediacy of video feedback, would have made it more difficult for the client to deny the connection between her physical appearance and her psychological issues.

Video feedback given outside the primary therapeutic relationship is a qualitatively different experience from when the feedback is given within the therapy session, but nonetheless it is potentially very valuable. Even under these circumstances, an overconcern for violating turf and thus diluting the transference between the client and the primary therapist seems unwarranted.

In general, this technique demonstrates how self-confrontation procedures can be employed effectively in confronting a client with a severe emotional difficulty, a manifestation of which is a distorted self-image. Although presenting a picture to a client of his or her body will not directly change that self-image, it is possible to use the picture as one among many methods within the context of psychotherapy to confront and explore relevant psychodynamics.

## Tourette's Syndrome

Chabot (1976) reported on his use of video techniques in the treatment of a child admitted to Sagamore Children's Center who was subsequently diagnosed as having Gilles de la Tourette syndrome. In the initial interview "Tommy" was observed having multiple motor tics of the face and extremities, and cursed frequently in an uncontrolled manner (coprolalia). The treatment plan included medication, parent counseling, and video sessions in order to help Tommy monitor and control his behavior. Brief, unstructured play sessions were video-taped. Both the therapist and Tommy together counted the frequency of Tommy's cursing during the feedback session, with the therapist helping to discriminate between the deliberate cursing and the cursing which was unintentional and a function of Tommy's involuntary vocal tic. Initially, Tommy was both embarrassed and surprised to see how often he cursed, twitched, and blinked. The video represented the first opportunity Tommy had to see himself the way others saw him. Chabot reports this self-confrontation as having a dramatic effect on Tommy. Besides the continued self-monitoring sessions, Tommy was also encouraged to become aware of his cursing through the use of a wrist counter which he wore all day long.

During the initial stages of treatment, Tommy cursed at the average rate of more than seven obscenities per minute. After two weeks with two video sessions per week, the cursing had diminished to a rate of one to two times in each half-hour session. Although it is obvious that this dramatic change could not have been attributed solely to the video sessions since Tommy was concurrently receiving a major tranquilizer, the video feedback did give Tommy the opportunity to monitor his own progress as well as increase his sense of awareness and self-control. Tommy's self-conscious embarrassment gradually diminished as he began to enjoy watching himself on TV, especially as he became increasingly free of the uncontrollable cursing which provoked both his parents and peers.

## Assertion Training

Most forms of training in assertiveness include such techniques as behavior rehearsal, instruction, coaching, discussion, homework assignments, and modeling. Videotape techniques are especially useful in those assertion training models which require behavioral rehearsal and modeling.

Several assertive training strategies utilizing video will be briefly outlined here. These were selected mostly for their heuristic value; a combination of elements from different approaches in a framework comfortable to the therapist would be the best way of utilizing the summaries to follow.

The approach taken by Galassi, Galassi, and Litz (1974) is a fairly comprehensive one and will be summarized first. Assertiveness training groups were led by male–female trainer teams. Two 90-minute sessions were conducted each week, and each session was divided into three half-hour segments. In the first segment, groups discussed the rationale for assertiveness, related readings, and the results of *in vivo* practice assignments that were given beforehand. They also learned to discriminate among assertive, nonassertive, and aggressive responses. During the second and third segments, groups viewed model videotapes of assertive interactions and then divided into dyads which practiced the modeled scenes repeatedly. The dyads also engaged in both directed and improvised roleplaying. Each dyad received peer, trainer, and/or video feedback on his or her performance during each session, including feedback on such variables as eye contact, appropriateness, and brevity of assertive statements, adequacy of delivery, and anxiety level. Practice situations were presented in increasing order of difficulty in order to minimize anxiety.

Situations rehearsed in the first four sessions involved only assertion toward members of the same sex, while the remaining sessions were concerned with opposite sex interactions. Galassi and co-workers report the general effectiveness of this approach on a variety of assertiveness measures. In ranking the importance of the ten components of the assertive training program in helping the subjects to modify their behavior, the subjects mentioned the video feedback aspect with trainer comments as first in importance. A follow-up report (Galassi, Kostka, & Galassi, 1975) noted that the positive effects of this treatment strategy remained one year later.

A methodology designed by Rathus (1973) capitalized on a combination of videotaped assertive models and directed practice. Groups of undergraduate women met once a week for seven weeks in hour-long sessions. These women were shown videotapes of women demographically similar discussing assertive behavior which included specific examples of assertiveness. Each tape included these women demonstrating specific examples of assertive behavior. At the conclusion of each session, group members were given homework assignments which necessitated recording the results of attempts at practicing the particular behaviors discussed on the videotape.

The method calls for demonstrating the following nine types of assertive behavior:

1.  Assertive talk (for example, "I was here first," "I'd like more coffee, please.")
2.  Feeling talk (for example, "I am so sick of that man.")
3.  Greeting talk (Smile brightly and say, "Hi! I haven't seen you in months!")
4.  Passively and actively disagreeing (Change the topic, look away, disagreeing actively when sure.)
5.  Asking why (Insist on explanations from authority figures.)
6.  Talking about oneself (Relate personal experiences.)
7.  Agreeing with compliments ("That's an awfully nice thing to say. I appreciate it.")
8.  Avoiding trying to justify opinions ("Are you always so disagreeable?")
9.  Looking people in the eye.

In each of the seven sessions, the group members were shown a videotape. The videotape shown in the first session consisted of Rathus explaining the nature of the nine types of assertive behaviors enumerated above. The videotape also included models who made comments and requested clarifications. The second videotape consisted of assertive models reconstructing their experiences using assertive, feeling, and greeting talk. The third tape showed the models talking about their experiences with passive and active disagreement, asking why, talking about themselves, and agreeing with compliments. In the fourth tape, the assertive models discussed their experiences, avoiding justifying their opinions to "habitually disputatious persons," and looking people in the eye. The fifth tape focused on the ways assertiveness may be used profitably with peers, relatives, and teachers, and in the sixth session the models discussed how assertiveness could be used with members of the opposite sex. In the last session a tape was shown of a question-and-answer session between the models and Rathus, dealing generally with advice to those who need help in social interactions.

This method was found to be more effective than both a placebo treatment and a nontreatment control in inducing assertiveness in undergraduate women. While Rathus does not use roleplaying in his model, this, along with constructive feedback, would be a likely addition to his program.

Most forms of assertive training that employ models use either live or audiotaped models. There are two advantages of using videotaped models. The first advantage is that the performance of the model could be carefully rehearsed until the performance contains all the elements of assertion that clients are expected to imitate. The second advantage is that it is possible to present each client with an identical stimulus which would not vary in any behavioral aspect; this would permit more valid comparisons among client responses to the procedure.

In a program very similar to that described in the parent training section, Curran and his colleagues (Curran & Gilbert, 1975; Curran, Gilbert, & Little, 1976) trained "date-anxious" subjects with instruction, discussion, videotape modeling, behavioral rehearsal, group and videotape feedback, homework assignments, and social reinforcement. These skills focused on: giving and receiving compliments; feeling talk; listening skills; assertion; nonverbal communication methods; ways of handling silence; training in planning and asking for dates; ways of enhancing physical attractiveness; and approaches to physical intimacy problems. Each weekly session focused on one or two of these skill areas.

Stimulus tapes (see Chapter 7, p. 138) are also useful in assertive training. For example, responses to certain interpersonal situations may be used for training assertive responses; the following sample scenes, used as part of a research project by Hersen, Eisler, and Miller (1974), can be effective in a clinical situation.

**Sample One.** *Narrator.* "You're in a crowded grocery store and in a hurry. You pick one small item and get in line to pay for it. You're really trying to hurry because you're already late for an appointment. Then, a woman with a shopping cart full of groceries cuts in line in front of you."

*Woman.* "You don't mind if I cut in here, do you? I'm in a hurry."

**Sample Two.** *Narrator.* "You take your car to a service station to have a grease job and the oil changed. The mechanic tells you that your car will be ready in an hour. When you return to the station you find that in addition to the oil change and grease job, they have given your car a major tune up."

*Cashier.* "That comes to $215. Will that be cash or charge?"

**Sample Three.** *Narrator.* "You have just bought a new shirt, and upon putting it on for the first time discover that several buttons are missing. You return to the store and approach the saleslady who sold it to you."

*Saleslady.* "May I help you?"

**Sample Four.** *Narrator.* "It is your only day off and you have several important errands to run. As you are leaving your house, your neighbor comes over and wants to borrow your car. You really need your car."

*Neighbor.* "How about letting me borrow your car for a while; I want to ride over to the drugstore and get a magazine."

**Sample Five.** *Narrator.* "You are at home alone watching your favorite television show when someone knocks on your door. When you open the door you find a woman who announces that she is selling vacuum cleaners."

*Woman.* "Let me come in and demonstrate our latest model. It will only take fifteen minutes of your time."

**Sample Six.**   *Narrator.* "As you arrive at work one morning you notice a woman employee pulling into the parking space assigned to you. You really cannot afford to be late this morning. The woman rolls down her window."

*Woman.* "Will it be okay if I park here?" (p. 298)

As was done in the research of Hersen and colleagues, a videotaped model may be instructed to respond assertively to each of these situations. The specific assertive behaviors which are to be taught in the group are rehearsed by the person who serves as the model. The videotape methodology permits redoing the modeling tape until the model "gets it right," that is, until it adequately portrays the elements of assertiveness to be taught. Afterward, these assertive behaviors can be instructed, modeled, roleplayed, and rehearsed.

## Parent Training

Parent training is an increasingly popular modality, both for its preventive value and for the therapeutic value it has for disturbed children and their families. In its popularity, multifarious combinations of techniques have been applied, each based on slightly different theoretical perspectives. Most programs utilize some or all of the following techniques: lectures, modeling, roleplaying, homework assignments, and behavior rehearsal. Several "canned" parent training books and programs are available for use by either parents alone or in conjunction with a formalized program led by a trained professional.

Those who have used video in conjunction with parent training programs typically report remarkable results, to the extent that Baker (1982, personal communication) called video "almost a necessity." Those who use video in training parents see it as an excellent way of reducing the time needed for training, increasing parents' abilities to see the consequences their behavior has on their children (and vice versa), and as a way of demonstrating improvement as parents learn new skills. One study reported that of the several techniques used in their parent training group, video feedback was viewed by the parents as the most beneficial (Durrett & Kelly, 1974).

What follows is a description of a model training program for individually training parents. Variations in this technique are encouraged, especially in order to tailor the program to both the individual and unique needs of the parent population and to the therapist's orientation. The core strategy of the technique described below was developed in 1968 by Dr. Martha Bernal and her colleagues at UCLA (Bernal, Duryee, Pruett, & Burns, 1968; Bernal, 1969).

Bernal and her associates use the term "brat behaviors" to describe the child who tantrums frequently, is assaultive, threatening, and defiant. Her program was devised specifically for use with parents of "brats." It is assumed that much of the undesirable behavior found in children with emotional difficulties is being maintained by the parents' behaviors. Therefore, the first step in the process of training parents individually is to assess the quality of the parent–child interaction. This can be done either at home or in a studio (or video-equipped office) at the site of the training program.

Step 1: Observation. Observation performed in the home has the advantage of being most like the situation to which trained behaviors are intended to generalize. The obvious difficulty with this technique is the time and personnel required to visit the home environment and to make videotapes of parent–child interaction. While it is certainly more authentic than seeing the interaction patterns in the office, home observation can also be artificial. In fact, it is clear that most of the vital patterns are just as clear when the parent or parents and child are asked to interact in a studio or office.

Step 2: Analysis. An analysis of the taped interaction provides a foundation for designing custom-tailored instructions to the parent, based on specific skills required for remediating specific deficits in the parent–child relationship. Frequently, when a parent learns to modify a specific behavior, this knowledge generalizes to similar behaviors in other situations.

Step 3: Instruction. The instruction phase is in actuality the core of treatment. Excerpts are played from the prior treatment session in order to demonstrate points in the replay at which certain skills need to be employed, or simply to help the parent identify these patterns. Parents are then given specific instructions for the videotaped interaction to follow. For example, parents may be taught to reduce verbalizations, selectively ignore the child's aversive behavior, establish specific behaviors as conditioned negative reinforcers, or identify acceptable behaviors and positively reinforce them through attention, praise and warmth. Playing of videotapes and instruction may last anywhere from 20 to 45 minutes, depending on the parent and the behaviors to be learned.

Step 4: Videotaped Interaction. Immediately following the instructions, parent and child are asked to engage in approximately 15 minutes of interaction, utilizing the newly learned skill.

Step 5: Immediate Feedback. When appropriate, parents should be reinforced positively for their success at accomplishing the assigned task. During this phase, parents can also be shown portions of the videotape just completed, and given feedback on how well they accomplished the task.

Prior to the next meeting, the tape made during Step 4 can be reviewed by the therapist in order to evaluate the parent's performance, and plan the following week's interventions.

This general treatment paradigm has been demonstrated to have significant effects in eliminating so-called brat behaviors and in increasing the degree of mutual affection between parent and child in as little as seven intervention or training sessions. (Bernal, 1968).

One advantage of this technique is that, because it is administered individually and is flexible, it is uniquely customized for use with specific problems held by specific individuals. This should increase the likelihood of success. One difficulty, however, is the extra time and/or staff required to train many clients in this manner. There are only certain types of parents and certain types of children who can benefit from such a program. Parents must have the ego strength to be able to examine their own behavior, and they must be open to criticism and feedback from the instructor/therapist. Cooperation is a necessity. Uncooperative relatives may also obstruct the process; in the event of a highly disturbed family system, parent training cannot substitute for family therapy. Although only one parent can be trained at a time in this program, training another parent as well could elicit greater cooperation. It must be emphasized that in order for this technique to be appropriate, the child must have a high enough rate of problem behaviors for the behaviors to be manifested in the videotaped interaction.

***Parents As Surrogate Therapists.***   Another, slight modification of this technique was accomplished by Furman and Feighner (1973) and Feighner and Feighner (1974). In the program at the Psychiatric Institute at Alvarado in San Diego, 15 to 20-minute parent–child interactions are videotaped and used immediately thereafter as a basis for discussing and teaching parents how to effectively employ behavioral strategies for coping with their child's behavior. In this program, parents are seen as surrogate therapists because they are taught behavioral principles which they are requested to implement at home with their children.

The stage is set by the therapist discussing and probing for some recent emotionally laden experience which could serve as a situation for on-camera interaction. The therapist then leaves the room and the parent and child interact before the camera. Feighner and her colleagues note that parents and child both seem to ignore the camera once the interaction begins. These brief sessions provide ample material for training and feedback purposes.

The child is then sent to a playroom while the parent and therapist review the session. Initially, observations tend to be directed toward the inevitably low occurrence of positive reinforcement. Positive reinforcement techniques are taught to the parents, and aversive measures are discouraged and recommended only in instances where the child is acting dangerously or destructively.

*Microtraining.* Durrett and Kelly (1974) used a microtraining format for their parent training groups, based on the communication skills outlined by Ivey (1971). These skills, although initially discussed in reference to the counselor–counselee relationship, can easily and fruitfully be applied to intrafamilial relationships. These behaviors include:

1. Attending Behavior: eye contact, body posture, verbal follow-up; open invitation to talk; minimal encouragement to talk
2. Listening Skills: Selective Attention: reflection and summarization of feeling; paraphrasing and summative paraphrase
3. Skills of Self-Expression: expression of feeling; expression of content; direct, mutual communication

The group met twice a week for only three weeks, but each session lasted two and a half hours. Each session consisted of: introducing a specific skill; discussing readings from a written manual; watching a videotape that modeled the specific skill; watching a portion of a videotape of an interview of a family member in the group made previously; producing a video made of couples practicing a new skill; reviewing this videotape with a group while focusing on the particular skill; and assigning homework consisting of rehearsing the newly acquired skill in specific home situations. Because of the large amount of material to be covered in two and a half hours, the authors recommend no more than eight people attend the group at one time.

*Review of Child's Psychotherapy Session.* Another interesting method of training parents to understand the behavior of their children is mentioned by Chabot (1976). With the child's explicit approval, parents observe videotape recordings of the child's therapy session. The therapist and the parent together discuss the child's motivations for his or her behavior using the videotape of the child's therapy session as the stimulus for discussion. This procedure helps parents to understand their child's motivations and gives them another paradigm for relating to their child. This is not to say that parents ought to act like therapists toward their children but that the kind of unconditional warmth delivered by the therapist may help the parent accept the child's behavior as being a result of the child's feelings, and thus able to understand that these feelings are acceptable. This also takes the mystery out of the therapy process for the parent (thus increasing cooperation) and removes the therapist from the dubious role of middleman. A technique which involves the parents serving as therapists is discussed earlier in this chapter.

***Start-Stop Procedures.***   This method of training uses a stimulus vignette as a basis for discussion of children's motivations for their behavior, and the effects that parental behaviors have on children (and vice-versa). The prototype of this method, developed by clinicians at the San Fernando Valley Child Guidance Clinic, presents a brief videotaped vignette showing a fairly common but problematic sequence of child behaviors (for example, an argument that erupts out of refusing to share a toy with a sibling, or disrupting a parent while the parent attempts to clean the house). Each vignette is discussed, and the parents are invited to comment on it and suggest possible interventions. Following this discussion, the parents are shown three or four videotaped interventions that are graded according to effectiveness and appropriateness. The videotape is stopped for a brief discussion following each intervention. These procedures can easily be combined with other techniques, such as roleplaying and behavior rehearsal, to offer a thorough approach to parent training. (The professionally produced stop-start videotape, along with a training manual, can be purchased by contacting Meg Caldwell, San Fernando Valley Child Guidance Clinic, 9650 Zelzah Ave., Northridge, Ca. 91325.)

***"Canned Programs."***   I have used video very successfully in the "confident parenting" approach as discussed by Eimers and Aitchison (1978). This empirically based program combines didactic material with modeling, roleplaying, rehearsal, and homework, and teaches parents to implement such interventions as effective praising, effective limit setting, time out, and ignoring. Videotaped models demonstrating the proper way to administer these interventions are particularly helpful to parents. Watching the videotaped models helps review the basic points of each technique. Each of the topics listed above is broken down into its components and demonstrated to the parent group who then roleplay with each other and then critique themselves on whether or not they were able to perform all components of each activity. For example, effective praising requires the implementation of the following seven components:

1. look at your child;
2. move close to your child;
3. smile;
4. say lots of nice things to your child;
5. praise behavior, not the child;
6. be physically affectionate;
7. praise the behavior immediately.

Examples of praise statements are given as well. The remaining interventions, for example, limit setting and mild social disapproval, are also taught by breaking them down into their components.

Videotape methodology can be used similarly in other canned programs, for example, Parent Effectiveness Training (Gordon, 1970) or Systematic Training for Effective Parenting (Dinkmeyer & McKay, 1976). Within these programs video can be used as a way of modeling the appropriate interventions as taught by the program, or in combination with roleplaying as a way of giving feedback to parents on how well they are learning and performing the tasks.

## Sex Therapy

Videotape has been used in a variety of different ways to treat sexual dysfunction. As an educative tool, video teaches new skills and clarifies misconceptions. As a result it also tends to allay anxiety and mitigate fears. The educative function also includes a modeling aspect in which clients are encouraged to emulate the skills demonstrated on the videotaped presentation. Video has also been used more directly in the treatment of sexual dysfunctions, as a source of feedback, and as a form of desensitization.

The effectiveness of education alone in the treatment of sexual dysfunction is highlighted by the research of Jankovich and Miller

(1978). They found that with no interventions other than an audiovisual sex education program, approximately 40 percent of their primarily anorgasmic research subjects became orgasmic within a week of viewing the program. Other research (Robinson, 1974) supports the value of videotaped materials as an educative component within a sex therapy program. McMullen (1976), however, found no differences between videotaped and booklet presentation of information about masturbation in treating primary orgasmic dysfunction. This raises the possibility that video mediated information about sexual dysfunction may be more helpful in treating sexual dysfunction that is a result of other difficulties. This prospect underlines the necessity of including other interventions in the treatment of sexual dysfunction, and perhaps more important, the need for further research into this area.

An example of an approach capitalizing on the modeling aspect was provided by Hartman and Fithian (1972) who showed clients films and photographs of research couples using "nondemand" coital techniques. They also used audiotapes of a woman describing how she became orgasmic and how she taught others to become orgasmic. Following this audiotape presentation, a videotape is shown of the same woman engaging in intercourse, as well as a videotape of the woman that she emulated becoming orgasmic.

There is some question about whether it is better to show videotapes of a model to a client before or after asking the client to perform desired activities. Some clinicians using this technique (for example, Renick, 1973) believe it is more appropriate to show to clients prior to engaging in the activity because this capitalizes on the modeling aspect of the process. Others (for example, More, 1973), however, prefer to show the client videotapes following the couple's attempts to engage in the prescribed activities in order to prevent performance anxiety.

An interesting program that made multiple uses of video occurred at the University of California School of Medicine in the Sex Advisory and Counseling Unit (S.A.C.U.). Among other aspects of this multifaceted service program, seminars were occasionally presented which consisted of two four-hour sessions, spaced a week apart. The first focused on female sexuality and the second on male sexuality. The men and women were segregated for the presentation and discussions. In the women's session, several female therapists presented material on anatomy and physiology, followed by discussions concerning such topics as sexual myths, performance anxieties, individual differences, sex-role stereotyping, and communicating one's sexual needs. While this occurred, the group of men watched the presentation on closed-circuit video in an adjoining room. The process was reversed the following week for the presentation on male sexuality. Vandervoort and Blank (1975) suggest that the effectiveness of this procedure rests in the fact that it allowed participants to interact more freely with the presenters without the tension caused by the immediate presence of their partners or members of the opposite sex. The modeling component of the presentation included the presentation of films of a woman masturbating to orgasm, a couple making love without intercourse, an abstract sensual film, and two brief films contrasting sex-as-fun with sex-as-work.

Both the permission-giving tone of the films and the openness of the panel contributed to the generally positive response to the sessions. Many participants felt that they were no longer in need of further counseling after attendance at these seminars.

The use of videotaped modeling procedures offers the advantage over reading material of being closer to reality. This advantage, however, must be weighed against the potential liability of videotaped sexual material; in its realistic portrayal of sexual activity, these videotapes may offend the sensitivities of some clients. While most sex therapists agree that education is an essential component in the treatment of sexual dysfunction, media should be used discriminately, taking into account the needs and values of the particular clients.

An interesting example of video used in treatment was provided by Serber (1974). In a special room, a microphone was placed on the floor near a bed to record the couple's verbal intercourse, while a camera with a wide-angle lens was placed approximately 12 feet away from the bed to record the couple's sexual intercourse. The couple had complete control over the videotape equipment and was given instructions on how to use the equipment. The videotape was brought into the therapy session and reviewed by the therapist who found that there were often large differences between what the couple had reported as occurring and what actually occurred in their lovemaking. Serber discovered that the video feedback helped to desensitize the couple to previously threatening, anxiety-provoking behavior. The playback session also motivated the couple to complete homework assignments in a more systematic fashion.

Prior to becoming involved in this form of treatment, the couples were informed of the method of treatment in detail, as well as of the rationale, and they signed consent forms agreeing to be videotaped. The couples also were informed that the videotape of their sexual activity would be in their possession and their property at all times. Most couples were amenable to this procedure. Both the facts that they were not being watched "live," and the thorough control they had over the presentation helped to ease their tension. The few clients who reported initial anxiety found that their anxiety shortly decreased. The chief advantages of this technique, according to Serber, were the fact that the therapist was better able to diagnose the areas in which the couple was having difficulty and the fact that the therapist was able to reinforce positive behaviors.

# 9

# Special Applications/Advanced Technology

The emphasis throughout this book has been on activities and techniques that could be used with a bare minimum of equipment: a camera, video recorder, and monitor (or TV set). This chapter will briefly describe some techniques possible with the addition of slightly more sophisticated equipment.

The simplest piece of additional equipment is a switching device which allows the use of more than one camera and the ability to shift from one to another while recording. Beyond this, the creative mixture of images from more than one camera is achieved by the use of a special-effects generator. This piece of equipment permits "wipes" (the change from one scene to another by a windshield wiperlike motion), dissolves, and superimpositions (overlaying one image on top of another). Special-effects generators also permit dividing the screen into quarters of adjustable proportion and allows different images to be shown in different quarters. When the screen is divided in order to accomplish this, one has achieved a "split-screen" effect. While special-effects generators were once beyond the budgets of individual users, they are now available for as little as $1500. If, however, you have access to a university or a well-equipped video studio, it is more than likely that you will have a special-effects generator available.

Another piece of equipment that you may find useful is the projection television. These are currently being marketed in well-stocked appliance stores for between two- and four-thousand dollars, and they permit watching video replays on an approximately 2½- by 3-foot screen. These are especially useful for stimulus tapes because the person on the screen to whom the client reacts is more lifelike in size.

Innovations in broadcast television production are not discussed in detail here because they are beyond the control of the individual practitioner. One example of a broadcast innovation that could have important therapeutic effects is "dual audio television" (Borton, 1971). This interesting innovation calls for a separate audio channel to be broadcast for children of different age groups. Through a separate transistor radio receiver, an announcer weaves commentary between the program's verbal script and music. This commentary is aimed at increasing the relevance of commercial television to children; it increases general knowledge, process knowledge, affective knowledge, and foreign language comprehension.

Another broadcast innovation currently being test-marketed in several cities is "interactive television" in which the television audience has the capability of making limited responses to inquiries delivered over the television set. While the therapeutic uses for such a procedure remain to be explored, it is likely that interactive television can be useful in the teaching of psychology.

This brief chapter also discusses such activities as interpersonal process recall that require the use of more than one camera and multi-image, immediate self-confrontation.

Although advanced technology increases the quality of what can be achieved technically, there is not yet a single piece of equipment that can substantially enhance the therapeutic value of self-confrontation achieved with the simplest of equipment. This is due to the fact that most of the therapeutic work is done by the therapist, not by the equipment. Nevertheless, those who wish to invest in more sophisticated equipment will most likely find the activities in this chapter enjoyable and effective.

## The Activities

### The Split-screen Technique

The split-screen technique in which the screen is divided into sections, each section portraying an image from a different camera, is most useful in group and family therapy. In these contexts the split-screen shows an individual speaking while simultaneously portraying the reactions of another individual or of the rest of the group.

One arrangement is to show the therapist in a corner of the screen while the group fills the remainder of the screen. This poses a problem because part of the group is inevitably lost in such an arrangement. Another technique is to use a corner "insert" of the group member who is talking while the rest of the group fills the screen; this, of course, does not change the problem of losing part of the group in the monitor. A third arrangement is to show a group member in the corner of a screen watching the replay of the group session that is being shown on the rest of the screen.

The split-screen technique can also be used in individual therapy and in supervision. In these cases the client is seen on one portion of the screen while the therapist is seen on another, thus bridging the distance gap and allowing simultaneous close-ups of both. In order to convey that the client is the primary subject, a full-face close-up can be used of the client while a side view may be used for the therapist. If two full-face images were being shown, the viewer would be distracted by trying to decide which to look at, thereby taking the attention away from the session itself.

A dramatic effect can be achieved by horizontally splitting the screen and placing a shot of the client's eyes above or below the therapist's eyes. Gaze directedness, eye contact, and variations in pupil size can be important cues to attitude, feeling, and even deception (Heilveil, 1976). The interaction of eye movements gives clues to the ongoing shifts in the transference–countertransference relationship.

## Interpersonal Process Recall

"Interpersonal process recall" is a technique developed by Kagan and his associates at Michigan State University in the early '60s and refined over a 15-year period. It is a complex technique that requires several staff members, split-screen capability, more than one room, and specialized training. A film package entitled "Influencing Human Interaction" which describes the use of IPR and can also be used to assist in training professionals in this technique* is available from Mason Media, Inc., Box C, Mason, Michigan, 48854.

Kagan's team observed that when a person is videotape recorded while engaging in psychotherapy (or counseling), the person is able to recall thoughts and feelings with extreme clarity when shown the

---

*Because of the complexity of IPR only a cursory review of the technique is provided here. The reader is referred to the following sources, as well as the training materials, for further information: Kagan, Schauble, Resnikoff, Danish, & Krathwohl, 1969; Resnikoff, Kagan, & Schauble, 1970; Archer & Kagan, 1973; Woody, Krathwohl, Kagan, & Farquhar, 1965; Kagan, Krathwohl, & Miller, 1963; Archer, Fiester, Kagan, Rate, Spierling, & Van Noord, 1972; and Spivack, 1974.

recording immediately afterward. When given the power to start and stop the recording at will, clients often pour forth with new and important insights that give them deeper understanding of their psychodynamics. This process could be facilitated to an even greater degree by allowing the person to view the videotape without the therapist present, but instead in the presence of a third person who encourages the client to explore various avenues related to the client's underlying motives.

At least two rooms are necessary for the IPR process, and a third is desirable. One room serves as a studio in which videotaping and recall sessions are held and the second room is equipped for viewing and recording recall sessions. A third room can be positioned so that the activities in the two other rooms can be observed through one-way mirrors. In the studio, two cameras are installed in corners, each focused on a chair facing the camera. When the interview is enacted the therapist's and client's heads and upper torsos are videotaped and enlarged as much as the monitor permits. A special-effects generator blends the two images so that they are relayed to a single monitor in a split-screen fashion.

In the first phase of the IPR session, therapist and client enter the studio and begin a standard psychotherapeutic interview. This interview is observed, either through a one-way mirror or on a monitor in an adjacent room by a third person who will serve as an "inquirer." (This person has also been called an "interrogator" and a "recall worker.") After the session is completed, the videotape is rewound for replay. The therapist and the client then adjourn to separate rooms. The inquirer joins the client to view a replay of the session while the therapist may also view the replay in a different room (perhaps the original studio where the initial interview was held).

The next step in the IPR process is the recall session, in which the original session just completed is replayed over the monitors. Either the client or the inquirer may start or stop the videotape machine at will through the use of a remote-control switch accessible to both.

The inquirer's function is to facilitate the client's self-analysis through gentle but assertive prodding aimed at disclosing underlying motivations, expectations, thoughts, and feelings, especially as they relate to the client's interaction with the therapist. The inquirer clearly does not attempt to establish a relationship similar to that of the therapist and client. This is discouraged by keeping the client focused chiefly on the feelings engendered in the replay, by commenting only on the transactions occurring between therapist and client, by reminding the client to concentrate only on the recall, and by prompting the client to focus attention on the monitor. In fact, Kagan and his colleagues once experimented with switching inquirers after every few sessions and found that this did not adversely effect the client's progress. Following the recall phase, the newfound knowledge gained from the recall worker is brought back to the next therapy session.

The best inquirers are often skilled clinicians, for they tend to be sensitive to the nuances that reveal conflicts. Yet the inquirer must limit probing to the immediate past. The importance of the third person doing the interrogating is underscored by the fact that most often therapists will avoid the same aspects of their behavior in the recall sessions as they did during the original session. Clients also are freer to express in the recall stage feelings they may have toward their therapist that they would be uncomfortable expressing directly in the therapist's presence. Inquirers must be concerned primarily with actively teaching clients how to interrogate themselves, and not as concerned with relating clients' behavior and feelings to feelings and actions outside of the session. The inquirer attempts to create within clients an intense awareness of their behavior in the client–therapist relationship, and to help clients enter into new, more healthy relationships with their therapists. In doing this, the inquirer encourages clients to discuss their likes and dislikes concerning their behavior with their therapist, as well as their feelings, thoughts, self-concepts, feelings about ways in which they would like their therapist to see them, and feelings about how their therapist actually does see them.

There are three variations on the recall phase of the technique: therapist alone, client alone, and therapist and client together (mutual recall). In the individual recalls, viewers examine dynamics which occur between viewer and partner during the original interaction, and the recall worker focuses on one of the partners (either the therapist or the client). In mutual recall, the two members of the dyad are confronted together by the recall worker; they are encouraged not only to discuss what occurred during the videotaped session but also to discuss their feelings in the "here and now."

IPR provides the subject with an abundance of material; this much information can flood the viewer. Viewers should therefore be gradually introduced to the process by a supportive person in the early stages of exposure.

There is evidence that the IPR process often dramatically accelerates the rate of a client's movement in counseling and psychotherapy. Clients are more willing to admit their discomfort, to commit themselves to the change process, to learn how to differentiate among their own feelings and environmental stimuli, and to change their behavior.

IPR has been used in a variety of applications. In psychotherapy, it has been used in conjunction with affect simulation (see Chapter 2, p. 21). In this merger of two video techniques, clients view an affect simulation vignette, prompting them to respond to affect-laden material. Clients are videotape recorded as they participate in the simulation. Following this, the clients engage in a recall session, in which the client explores his or her feelings during the simulation.

Another strategy combined the image of a client with a simultaneous recording of such physiological measures as galvanic skin response, heart rate, and eccrine sweat rate during a therapy session. The graphic output of these measures are videotaped concurrently and replayed in a split-screen format. Discussion then centers on those topics that are specifically stressful or anxiety provoking. Archer and co-workers (1972) combined the use of a stimulus film with this procedure. Three cameras were used, one focused on the film, the second on the client, and the third on the graphic output of the physiological measures. This, combined into a split-screen format, was replayed for the client within the context of an IPR recall session. Recall workers stopped the videotape whenever they noticed a significant increase in autonomic responsiveness. The client's feelings during these moments were then discussed.

Another variation of the technique is to combine it with hypnosis. Woody and his colleagues (1965) reported success at videotaping a counseling session followed by a recall session in which a recall worker viewed the videotapes of the counseling session; this recall session was also videotaped. Finally, a third session occurred in which the videotape of the recall session was analyzed by the original therapist and the client together. Hypnotic suggestions were given at the end of the regular session with the therapist and were aimed at increasing the client's sensitivity to cues while watching the videotape; achieving satisfaction from performing well in the IPR procedure; enhancing the ability to verbalize feelings, thoughts, attitudes, and emotions; and having positive reactions toward the recall worker.

## The Videoscan Technique

"Videoscan" is an acronym for "videotape self-confrontation after narcotherapy," and that is precisely what it is. Metzner (1978) devised this activity which involves videotaping a patient after injecting him or her with a hypnotic drug (usually sodium amobarbital or sodium thiopenthal), then replaying the interview when the patient is no longer under the influence of this mind-altering chemical. This combination of narcotherapy and self-confrontation helps a client to gain insight because the taped replays of the drug interviews usually contain material which the patient has repressed or suppressed.

During the narcotherapy interview the patient is usually better able to remember and discuss emotional material than the patient would have available without the medication. Occasionally patients will abreact traumatic events while under the influence, but more often they are simply less inhibited. Patients usually forget much of what happened during the narcotherapy session after the medication has worn off. Videotape is used essentially to help remind them. Rather than the therapist prodding the patient to remember, patients have the means to learn for themselves what occurred during the session. They are then assisted in integrating the material into consciousness by systematically scanning the contents of the videotape under the close guidance of the therapist.

Metzner lists four significant indications for the use of the videoscan technique. These include:

1. maladaptive neurotic, psychosomatic, and characterological symptoms, for example: amnesia; fugue states; conversion reactions; multiple personality; depression; anxiety states; bronchial asthma; and alcoholism;
2. unresolved diagnostic questions relating to the presence of repressed or inhibited psychological contents;
3. resistance to traditional psychiatric treatment approaches, for example, insight-oriented psychotherapy or hypnotherapy;
4. legitimate need on the part of the patient for more rapid alleviation of symptoms than had been provided by previous therapies.

Following are significant contraindications for videoscan:

1. psychotic or paranoid trends;
2. history of barbiturate hypersensitivity, porphyria, or chronic cardiac, renal or hepatic disease;
3. acute systemic illness.

The biggest problem with this technique is the fact that only a highly qualified physician can conduct this procedure. Because of the uncommon but potential complications of both video self-confrontation and narcotherapy, I recommend that the videoscan technique be attempted only with great care and only by psychiatrists who have thoroughly familiarized themselves with the methods that comprise it.

## Stereo TV

The use of more than one monitor and more than one camera for simultaneously feeding back a client's self-image helps clients, individually or in a group, to experience feedback from multiple sources. Since no one angle is de facto a true representation of a person, the use of multiple monitors gives a person the opportunity to choose the perspective that is most useful.

Such a procedure magnifies the quantity of information observed by the client. Berger (1978), for example, operates two cameras with four monitors. The four monitors and cameras can be positioned to maximize the degree of simultaneous feedback. The client can see a full view of him or herself while talking to the therapist. The client can also observe his or her face, hand and/or body movements while talking.

Clients can be asked to observe whether or not their facial and body expressions are congruent with their verbalizations and their feelings and to share with the therapist any indications of incongruity that the client may observe. Clients can also be told to be on the lookout for expressions or movements that seem to be characteristic of someone else they might know.

This sort of high intensity self-confrontation is useful for many clients but should be used cautiously with clients who are suicidal or with those whose self-hatred is firmly based in their body image.

Large groups typically pose problems because the necessary clarity is difficult to obtain when so many people must be squeezed into a small viewing area. This is also a problem with the split-screen technique; there is only so much that can be done when attempting to portray a large group in a small part of the screen.

One solution, devised by Wilmer (1968), is to use at least two cameras, placing one camera on each side of the group and recording simultaneously on two separate videotape recorders. A unidirectional microphone can also be aimed at each half of the group. The recordings are then replayed, side by side, giving stereo sound effects, as well as "stereo" visual effects.

The experience may be somewhat confusing at first, not knowing on which monitor to focus. After a time, however, the "tennis match" problem of switching from one monitor to another gives way to a rewarding totality and provides an absorbing experience. The limitations of this technique are set only by the expenditure of time, money, and effort given to the task or to recreating moments in time. A group of six can have a camera focused on each member, each with a lavalier microphone. In replay, six individual monitors can be placed around each other, with each group member in control of his or her own monitor. It is questionable whether the results of such an enormous undertaking would be worth the energy involved, but it does provide interesting food for thought.

## Superimposition

Superimposition is a technique that permits one image to be overlayed on another in such a fashion that both images are visible together, an effect easily obtained through the use of a special-effects generator.

This technique can be used with forceful effect in group and family therapy applications, in which the face of one group member can be superimposed on the image of the remainder of the group. The face of a family member who holds a prominent influential position in relation to the rest of the family can be superimposed on the remainder of the family in a way that powerfully illustrates the control this family member exerts on the others. Furthermore, the facial expression of this family member may also illustrate the mood of the entire group, or may show in counterpoint the degree to which an individual family member may be alone or in opposition to the rest of the family. It also serves as a symbol for one of the perceptual styles required of a therapist—to see and hear one person clearly while simultaneously attending to the other group members.

## Multi-image Immediate Impact Self-confrontation

The goal of this technique, developed by Berger in 1972 (Berger, 1978), is to bring about abreactive or cathartic discharge by helping the client get in touch with deeply repressed identifications and introjects. This is accomplished by confronting the client with a series of varying and distorted images of him or herself in a "tunnel effect" on the video monitor.

The equipment needed for this technique is a videotape recorder, two mobile cameras with zoom lenses, two monitors, one split-screen special-effects generator, and one or more microphones. One camera is focused on the client's face as the client either faces the therapist or looks away. With the split-screen special-effects generator and one camera with a zoom lens, the picture of the client's face (or part of it) is enlarged and placed to one side of the monitor, occupying between one third and one quarter of the monitor screen. The second camera is aimed at the picture on the monitor, causing the monitor to be filled with repeated images of the face, one image echoing another in what appears to be a near endless chamber of mirrors. The number of images can be controlled by turning the focus slowly on the second camera. This creates intriguing effects which either the client or therapist may wish to hold in order to discuss further. By opening or closing the lens aperture and thus letting in varying degrees of light, certain images are faded.

Multiple images move in series to either the right or left and become increasingly blurred the greater their distance from the original image; this original image remains clear as it is seen through the lens of the first camera.

The client has the choice of dealing with these images in three ways. The client can see and react spontaneously to the immediate impact of the closed-circuit images as they are being created; the client can react during the videotaped replay of the videotaped segments; or the client may respond both times. This last choice permits a comparison to be made between the associations made at the time of the taping and at the time of replay.

The multi-image effect can also be created without the aid of a special-effects generator, with just one monitor and one camera. This is difficult and requires careful positioning of the client and monitor; the therapist who does not have the extra equipment may wish to take time to perfect this technique before attempting it with a client.

Initial reactions to experiencing the clear and distorted images is one of interest or excitement. It carries with it the message that we are each composed of many different layers, some of which are more accessible and "in focus" than others. The client is encouraged to ventilate reactions to experiencing him or herself being distorted, fading away, and disappearing on the monitor. Berger notes that the most important aspect of this technique is not the concurrent reproduction of multiple self-images, but rather the fact that images are reproduced and created in tandem and are increasingly distorted, one after the other, and that this is contrasted with a clear image. Berger also believes that experiencing these multiple images can lead to a client's acceptance of the fact that he or she is fluid, and that his or her various self-concepts co-exist alongside either in both conflict and harmony.

These shadowlike presentations are not known, nor are they typically approved of, in daily consciousness. This stimulates the client to bring up associations to deeper aspects of the self, associations which may be seen by the client as the instant emergence of the "bad self."

Berger noted that of 40 clients who used this technique, all but one had highly significant free associations, that is, associations that were useful in working through significant issues. No harmful effects of the procedure were noted.

# Epilogue

Writing this book represented a journey, of sorts, for me. I began my work with video as a "resistant therapist," with some of the same objections discussed in the Introduction. Trained in a rather traditional model of psychodynamic psychotherapy, I was reluctant to bring anything into the therapeutic relationship that might encroach upon the most vital therapeutic elements—my client and myself. So I began my first use of video in therapy groups with adolescents. I expanded it then to the therapeutic classroom, and then to individual therapy with children. By that point, I had no difficulty getting excited about its uses in other forms of psychotherapy.

In putting together this book, I was interested in sharing with professionals and students the techniques that proved most helpful to me. In the process of writing it, I discovered some of the ways other professionals had incorporated video into their work, and hence improved my own skills. In trying the newer techniques, I found myself constantly adapting them to the specific demands of my own therapeutic work. I hope the reader finds him- or herself in a similar process, using the techniques discussed here as a springboard for ideas that are particularly useful to the demands of each new therapeutic challenge.

As the more than one hundred techniques in this book exemplify, video can assist the creative psychotherapist in a variety of ways. While I tried to incorporate those techniques that seemed practical to the clinician, there are other uses which were excluded due to their low applicability; Bahnson's work with multiple personality is a good example (see Berger, 1978). If you work with a highly specialized population, it is very possible that video technology may assist you in some ways not mentioned in this book. As I often tell my clients, it is the spirit of sensitive experimentation that makes for growth.

This book was designed to be used as a handbook—an easy reference tool that highlights the practical uses of video technology. As such, theoretical issues were only touched on lightly in the first chapter and in the overviews at the beginning of each subsequent chapter. If, however, you have decided to try some of the activities discussed in this book, you may have personally seen how they can help clients confront their idealized self-image, resulting in a better match between self-perceptions and others' views. You may have also seen video function as an aid to cutting through denial systems, raising self-expectations, defeating compulsions to repeat habitual self-defeating patterns, catalyzing identifications, working through conflicts, and triggering affect, associations, and insights. You may also have witnessed a democratization of the therapeutic relationship, and/or an enhanced mutuality between therapist and client. For more substantive discussions of theoretical issues, the reader is referred to the bibliography and references, where a substantial list of theoretical information can be found.

Sophisticated technology is increasingly becoming an intricate part of human ecology. While physicians depend on highly technical instruments in nearly all phases of diagnosis and treatment, there is often a reluctance among mental health practitioners to incorporate useful technology in a similar fashion. As our culture advances, we have the choice of embracing the new technology or hiding from it. We cannot escape it, nor do I believe that we should use it just because it is there; I do believe that if it helps us to do what we set out to do better, then it behooves us to continue to experiment with it and refine our techniques.

For those readers new to the use of video, it is hoped that this book helped introduce you to the many and diverse ways video can fruitfully be incorporated into the therapeutic process. For the already initiated, I hope that this book has provided you with some new perspectives and methods with which to approach your therapeutic endeavors. In either case, I welcome your suggestions and reactions.

# Appendix

This appendix contains lists of various sources that may be useful in your work with video as a therapeutic tool.

## Scripts

The following organizations provide scripts of noteworthy programs for nonprofit use. (See "Script Reading" in Chapter 5.)

The CBS Reading Program
51 West 52nd Street
New York, NY 10019

The Television Reading Program
Capital Cities Communications, Inc.
4100 City Line Avenue
Philadelphia, PA 19131

Movie Scriptreader Program
Films, Inc.
Moviestrip Division
1144 Wilmette Avenue
Wilmette, IL 60091

Scholastic Book Services
904 Sylvan Avenue
Englewood Cliffs, NJ 07632

The Semit Corporation
Research and Development in Education
The Times Publishing Company
St. Petersburg, FL  33702

Scriptskills
Universal Education and Visual Arts
Universal City Studios
Universal City, CA  91608

## Educational TV

There is a wide variety of programs available at low or no cost to
nonprofit mental health or educational settings. These are typically
instructional in nature, although there are some that can be used as
motivators for reading, writing, and social studies experiences. The
following agencies distribute these programs and will make a list of
their holdings available by request:

Agency for Instructional Television
Box A
Bloomington, IN  47401

Great Plains National Instructional Television Library
Box 80669
Lincoln, NE  68501

International ITV Co-op
Skyline Center
Suite 1207
5205 Leesburg Pike
Falls Church, VA  22041

## Intelligent Television

The activities in this book are not intended in any way to foster or
encourage the viewing of commercial television by children. The
negative effects of viewing commercial television on children are well-
documented. Many parents find themselves at a loss in intelligently
guiding their children through the maze of children's programming.
There are several organizations that have formed as advocacy groups to
improve the terrible state of children's programming. These groups
also provide information useful to parents in a variety of ways.

Action for Children's Television
46 Austin Street
Newtonville, MA  02160

PTA TV Action Center
700 North Rush Street
Chicago, IL  60611

Institute for Visual Learning
1061 Brooks Avenue
St. Paul, MN  55113

American Academy of Pediatrics
Box 1034
Evanston, IL  60204

The United States Government provided grants to four firms, totalling
nearly one million dollars, to prepare and test educational materials
designed to develop critical viewing skills in students. These materials
may be useful in a family therapy or parent counseling context. The
elementary school materials were prepared by Southwest Educational
Development Laboratory. Information about these materials may be
obtained from:

Learning and Media Research
SEDL
211 East 7th
Austin, TX  78701

Materials for middle-school-aged students may be obtained by
writing:

Educational Broadcasting Corporation
WNET, Channel 13
356 West 58th Street
New York, NY  10019

## Videotapes

There are literally hundreds, if not thousands, of videotapes available
for the teaching of various aspects of mental health to professionals and
the public alike. Professionally produced videotapes are available in
nearly every imaginable aspect of mental health. The best source
available is the *Health Sciences Video Directory* edited by Eidelberg
(1977). This book lists thousands of videotapes in the health sciences,

along with a description of each tape, its price, and where it may be obtained. It is oriented toward medicine, but it does include a generous listing of tapes available in the mental health field.

Other excellent sources for videotapes in mental health include the following:*

Carousel Films, Inc.
1501 Broadway
New York, NY 10036

Focus International, Inc.
505 West End Avenue
New York, NY 10024
(tapes on human sexuality)

CRM McGraw-Hill Films
Del Mar, CA 92014
(videotapes on human values, especially as they relate to children and adolescents)

National Institute of Mental Health
NIMH Drug Abuse Film Collection
National Audiovisual Center (GSA)
Washington, DC 20409
(videotapes on drug abuse)

National Institute of Mental Health
Catalog: Selected Mental Health Audiovisuals
5600 Fishers Lane
Rockville, MD 20852
(This is a catalogue; DHEW Publication No. (ADM) 76-259, 1975.)

Polymorph Films
331 Newbury Street
Boston, MA 02115
(tapes on parenting and children)

The Public Television Library
Video Program Service
475 L'Enfant Plaza West, S.W.
Washington, DC 20024

---

*Dr. Nancy Roeske of the University of Indiana School of Medicine provided me with the most current sources of instructional videotapes.

Time Life Multimedia
100 Eisenhower Drive
Paramus, NJ 07652

Audiovisual Center
Indiana University
Student Service 0001
Bloomington, IN 47401
(catalogue on sexuality, growth, and development)

Dr. Jerome L. Schulman
Director of Child Psychiatry
Children's Memorial Hospital
Chicago, IL
(excellent tapes on children)

High Scope Educational Research Foundation
600 North River Street
Ypsilanti, MI 48107
(Piaget videotapes)

Pharmaceutical companies also have a wide variety of films and videotapes available either for loan or rental. Those companies that loan audiovisual materials include Abbott, Ciba, Geigy, Lederle, Merrell, Roche, Roerig, Sandoz, Smith Kline & French, Squibb, and Upjohn. The Sandoz Film Library Geriatric videotapes are excellent, and may be obtained by writing:

Mr. H. L. Walther
Sandoz Pharmaceuticals
East Hanover, NJ 07936

Large universities, especially those with schools of medicine, maintain a listing of videotapes that may be loaned to individuals, educational institutions, or clinics. Research librarians at these facilities will answer questions on how to obtain such a list.

# References and Bibliography

Adams, V. Videotherapy. *Time*, 1973 (Feb. 26), 58.

Adler, L. M., Ware, J. E. and Enelow, A. J. Changes in medical interviewing style after instruction with two closed-circuit television techniques. *Journal of Medical Education*, 1970, 45, 21–28.

Alger, I. Freeze-frame video in psychotherapy. In Berger, M. M. (Ed.) *Videotape Techniques in Psychiatric Training and Treatment* (Second Edition). New York: Brunner/Mazel, 1978.

Alger, I. Audio-visual techniques in family therapy. *Seminars in Psychiatry*, 1973, 5, 185–193.

Alger, I. Therapeutic use of videotape playback. *Journal of Nervous and Mental Disease*, 1969, 148, 430–436.

Alger, I. and Hogan, P. Enduring effects of V–T playback experience on family and marital relationships. *American Journal of Orthopsychiatry*, 1969, 39(1), 86–89.

Alger, I. and Hogan, P. The use of videotape recordings in conjoint marital therapy. *American Journal of Psychiatry*, 1967a, 123(11), 1425–1429.

Alger, I. and Hogan, P. The impact of videotape recording on involvement in group therapy. *Journal of Psychoanalysis in Groups*, 1967b, 2(1), 50–56.

Alkire, A. and Brunse, J. Impact and possible casualty from videotape feedback in marital therapy. *Journal of Consulting and Clinical Psychology*, 1974, 42, 203–210.

Alley, J. M. The effect of self-analysis of videotapes on selected competencies of music therapy majors. *Journal of Music Therapy*, 1980, 17(3), 113–132.

Annon, J. S. and Robinson, C. H. Video in sex therapy. In Fryrear, J. L. and Fleshman, B. (Eds.) *Videotherapy in Mental Health*. Springfield, Ill.: Charles C Thomas, 1981.

Archer, J., Jr., Fiester, T., Kagan, N., Rate, L., Spierling, T. and Van Noord, R. New method for education, treatment, research in human interaction. *Journal of Counseling Psychology*, 1972, 19(4), 275–281.

Archer, J. and Kagan, N. Teaching interpersonal relationship skills on campus: A pyramid approach. *Journal of Counseling Psychology*, 1973, 20, 535–540.

Bahnson, C. B. Body and self-images associated with audio-visual confrontation. *Journal of Nervous and Mental Disease.* 1969, 148, 262–280.

Bailey, K. and Sowder, T. Audiotape and videotape self-confrontation in psychotherapy. *Psychological Bulletin*, 1970, 74, 127–137.

Baker, B. L. Personal communication, 1982.

Baker, T. B., Udin, H. and Vogler, R. E. The effects of videotaped modeling and self-confrontation on the drinking behavior of alcoholics. *International Journal of the Addictions*, 1975, 10, 779–793.

Bandura, A. *Principles of Behavior Modification.* New York: Holt, Rinehart and Winston, Inc., 1969.

Bandura, A. and Barab, P. Processes governing disinhibitory effects through symbolic modeling. *Journal of Abnormal Psychology*, 1973, 82, 1–9.

Barber, T. X. and Calverley, D. Comparative effects on "hypnotic-like" suggestibility of recorded and spoken suggestions. *Journal of Consulting Psychology*, 1964, 28, 384.

Barnes, L. H. and Pilowsky, I. Psychiatric patients and closed-circuit TV teaching: A study of their reactions. *British Journal of Medical Education*, 1969, 3, 58–61.

Bazuin, C. H. and Yonke, A. M. What and how to teach in a primary care setting. *Journal of Medical Education.* 1980, 55, 874–876.

Bean, B. W. and Duff, J. L. The effects of videotape and of situational and generalized focus of control upon hypnotic susceptibility. *American Journal of Clinical Hypnosis*, 1975, 18, 28–33.

Beck, T. K. Videotaped scenes for desensitization of test anxiety. *Journal of Behavior Therapy and Experimental Psychiatry*, 1972, 3, 195–197.

Benschoter, R. A., Wittson, C. L. and Ingham, C. G. Teaching and consultation by television. *Mental Hospitals*, 1965, 16(3), 99–104.

Berger, M. M. (Ed.) *Videotape Techniques in Psychiatric Training and Treatment* (Second Edition). New York: Brunner/Mazel, 1978.

Berger, M. M. (Ed.) *Videotape Techniques in Psychiatric Training and Treatment* (First Edition). New York: Brunner/Mazel, 1970.

Bernal, M. E. Behavioral feedback in the modification of brat behaviors. *Journal of Nervous and Mental Disease*, 1969, 148, 375–385.

Bernal, M. E., Duryee, J. S., Pruett, H. L. and Burns, B. J. Behavior modification and the brat syndrome. *Journal of Consulting and Clinical Psychology*, 1968, 32, 447–455.

Bodin, A. M. The use of videotapes. In A. Ferber et al. (Eds.) *The Book of Family Therapy.* New York: Science House, 1972.

Bodin, A. M. Videotape applications in training family therapists. *Journal of Nervous and Mental Disease*, 1969, 148, 251–261.

Borton, T. Dual audio television. *Harvard Educational Review*, 1971, 41, 64–78.

Boyd, H. S. and Sisney, V. V. Immediate self-image confrontation and changes in self-concept. *Journal of Consulting Psychology*, 1967, 31, 291–294.

Brooks, D. D. Teletherapy or how to use videotape feedback to enhance group process. *Perspectives in Psychiatric Care*, 1976, 14, 83–87.

Bryer, J. E. Video pen pals say "aloha." *Learning*, 1975 (Dec.), 22–24.

Byrne, D. Repression-sensitization as a dimension of personality. In B. A. Maher (Ed.), *Progress in Experimental Personality Research* (Vol. 1), New York: Academic Press, 1964.

Carrere, J. Le psycho cinematographie. Principes et technique. Application au traitement des malades convalescents de delirium tremens. *Annales Medico-Psychologiques*, 1954, 112, 240–245.

Chabot, J. A. Videotape techniques in child therapy: "One picture is worth a thousand words." Unpublished paper presented at the Twenty-eighth Annual Meeting of the American Association of Psychiatric Services for Children, San Francisco, Ca., 1976.

Cheyney, A. B. and Potter, R. L. *Video: A Handbook Showing the Use of the Television in the Elementary Classroom.* Stevensville, Mi.: Educational Service, Inc., 1980.

Chodoff, P. Supervision of psychotherapy with videotape: Pros and cons. *American Journal of Psychiatry*, 1972, 128, 810–823.

Chotzen, Y. E. and King, S. S. Misdemeanor: Case study of a videotape. *Audiovisual Instruction*, 1977 (Mar.), 54–55.

Cornelison, F. S. Samples of psychopathology from studies of self-image experience. *Diseases of the Nervous System*, 1963, 24 (4), 133–139.

Cornelison, F. S. and Arsenian, J. A study of the response of psychotic patients to photographing self-image experience. *Psychiatric Quarterly*, 1960, 34, 1–8.

Cornelison, F. S., Ruhe, D. S. and Polatin, P. Use of motion pictures for the teaching of psychiatry. In Nichtenhauser, Coleman, Ruhe (Eds.) *Films in Psychiatry, Psychology, and Mental Health.* New York: Health Education Council, 1953, 37–43.

Cornelison, F. S. and Tausig, T. N. A study of the self-image experience using videotape at Delaware State Hospital. *Delaware Medical Journal*, 1964, 36(11), 229–231.

Creer, T. L. and Miklich, D. R. The application of a self-monitoring procedure to modify inappropriate behavior: A preliminary report. *Behaviour Research and Therapy*, 1970, 8, 91–92.

Curran, J. P. Social skills training and systematic desensitization in reducing dating anxiety. *Behaviour Research and Therapy*, 1975, 13, 65–68.

Curran, J. P. and Gilbert, F. S. A test of the relative effectiveness of a systematic desensitization program and an interpersonal skills training program with date anxious subjects. *Behavior Therapy*, 1975, 23, 510–521.

Curran, J. P., Gilbert, F. S. and Little, L. M. A comparison between behavioral replication training and sensitivity training approaches to heterosexual dating anxiety. *Journal of Consulting and Clinical Psychology*, 1976, 23, 190–196.

Cutter, F. Psychological application of video equipment in group process. In Fryrear, J. L. and Fleshman, B. (Eds.) *Videotherapy in Mental Health*. Springfield, Ill.: Charles C Thomas, 1981.

Czajkoski, E. J. The use of videotape recordings to facilitate the group therapy process. *International Journal of Group Psychotherapy*, 1968, 18, 516–524.

Daitzman, R. J. Methods of self-confrontation in family therapy. *Journal of Marriage and Family Counseling*, 1977, 3(4), 3–9.

Danet, B. N. Impact of audio-visual feedback on group psychotherapy. *Journal of Consulting and Clinical Psychotherapy*, 1969a, 33, 632.

Danet, B. N. Videotape playback as a therapeutic device in group psychotherapy. *International Journal of Group Psychotherapy*, 1969b, 19, 433–440.

Danet, B. N. Self-confrontation in psychotherapy reviewed: Videotape playback as a clinical and research tool. *American Journal of Psychotherapy*, 1968, 22, 246–257.

Davis, R. A. The impact of self-modeling on problem behaviors in school-age children. *School Psychology Digest*, 1979 8(1), 128–132.

Day, L. and Reznikoff, M. Preparation of children and parents for treatment at a children's psychiatric clinic through videotaped modeling. *Journal of Consulting and Clinical Psychology*, 1980, 30(2), 213–227.

Denney, D. R. and Sullivan, B. J. Desensitization and modeling treatments of spider fear using two types of scenes. *Journal of Consulting and Clinical Psychology*, 1976, 44, 573–579.

DeVoe, M. W. and Sherman, T. M. A microtechnology for teaching prosocial behavior to children. *Child Study Journal*, 1978, 8(2), 83–91.

Dinkmeyer, D. and McKay, G. D. *Systematic Training for Effective Parenting: Parent's Handbook*. Circle Pines, Minn.: American Guidance Service, Inc., 1976.

Doyle, P. H. Behavior rehearsal to videotape simulations: Applications, techniques, and outcomes. In Fryrear, J. L. and Fleshman, B. (Eds.) *Videotherapy in Mental Health*. Springfield, Ill.: Charles C Thomas, 1981.

Dowrick, P. W. Suggestions for the use of edited video replay in training behavioral skills. *Journal of Practical Approaches to Developmental Handicap*, 1978, 2, 21–24.

Dowrick, P. W. and Raeburn, J. M. Video editing and medication to produce a therapeutic self model. *Journal of Consulting and Clinical Psychology*, 1977, 45(6), 1156–1158.

Durrett, D. D. and Kelly, P. A. Can you really talk with your child? A parental training program in communication skills towards the improvement of parent–child interactions. *Group Psychotherapy and Psychodrama*, 1974, 27, 98–109.

Eidelberg, L. (Ed.) *Health Sciences Video Directory*, New York: Shelter Books, Inc., 1977.

Eimers, R. and Aitchison, R. *Effective Parents/Responsible Children.* New York: McGraw-Hill, 1978.

Eisler, R. M., Hersen, M. and Agras, W. S. Effects of videotape and instructional feedback on nonverbal marital interaction: An analog study. *Behavior Therapy*, 1973a, 4, 551–558.

Eisler, R. M., Hersen, M. and Agras, W. S. Videotape: A method for the controlled observation of nonverbal interpersonal behavior. *Behavior Therapy*, 1973b, 4, 420–425.

Eisler, R. M., Hersen, M. and Miller, P. M. Effects of modeling on components of assertive behavior. *Journal of Behavior Therapy and Experimental Psychiatry*, 1973, 4, 1–6.

Eisler, R. M., Hersen, M. and Miller, P. M. Shaping components of assertive behavior with instructions and feedback. *American Journal of Psychiatry*, 1974, 131, 1344–1347.

Elias-Burger, S., Sigelman, C. K., Danley, W. E. and Burger, D. L. Teaching interview skills to mentally retarded persons. *American Journal of Mental Deficiency*, 1981, 85 (6), 655–657.

Ellis, A. and Grieger, R. *Handbook of Rational–Emotive Therapy.* New York: Springer Publishing Co., 1977.

Emery, J. R. and Krumboltz, J. O. Standard vs. individualized hierarchies in desensitization to reduce test anxiety. *Journal of Counseling Psychology*, 1967, 14, 204–209.

Emmitt, T. Institutional closed-circuit television. In Fryrear, J. L. and Fleshman, B. (Eds.) *Videotherapy in Mental Health.* Springfield, Ill.: Charles C Thomas, 1981.

Esveldt, K. C., Dawson, P. C. and Fornss, S. R. Effect of videotape feedback on children's classroom behavior. *Journal of Educational Research*, 1974, 67, 453–456.

Evans, R. and Clifford, A. Captured for consideration—Using videotape as an aid to the treatment of the disturbed child. *Child: Care, Health and Development*, 1976, 2, 129–137.

Faia, C. and Shean, G. Using videotape and group discussion in treatment of male chronic alcoholics. *Hospital and Community Psychiatry*, 1976, 27, 847–851.

Feighner, A. C. and Feighner, J. P. Multimodality treatment of the hyperkinetic child. *American Journal of Psychiatry*, 1974, 131, 459–463.

Feinstein, C. and Tamerin, J. S. Induced intoxication and videotape feedback in alcoholism treatment. *Quarterly Journal of Studies on Alcoholism.* 1972, 33, 408–416.

Feldman, R. G. and Paul, N. L. Identity of emotional triggers in epilepsy. *The*

*Journal of Nervous and Mental Disease*, 1976, 162(5), 345–353.

Folsom, C. H., Jr. and Grant, C. O. Crisis intervention: A model workshop. *Journal of College Student Personnel*, 1978, 19(4), 331–336.

Forrest, D. V., Ryan, H., Glavin, R. and Merritt, H. H. Through the viewing tube: Videocassette psychiatry. *American Journal of Psychiatry*, 1974, 131, 90–94.

Froelich, R. E. Learning via videotape simulation. In Berger, M. M. (Ed.) *Videotape Techniques in Psychiatric Training and Treatment* (Second Edition). New York: Brunner/Mazel, 1978.

Froelich, R. E. and Bishop, F. M. One plus one equals three. *Medical and Biological Illustration*, 1969, 19, 15–18.

Fryrear, J. L. and Fleshman, B. (Eds.) *Videotherapy in Mental Health*. Springfield, Ill.: Charles C Thomas, 1981.

Fuller, F. and Manning, B. A. Self-confrontation reviewed: A conceptualization for video playback in teacher education. *Review of Educational Research*, 1973, 469–528.

Furman, S. and Feighner, A. Video feedback in treating hyperkinetic children: A preliminary report. *American Journal of Psychiatry*, 1973, 130, 792–796.

Galassi, J. P., Kostka, M. D. and Galassi, M. D. Assertive training: A one year video feedback. *Journal of Counseling Psychology*, 1974, 21(5), 390–394.

Galassi, J. P., Kostka, M. D. and Galassi, M. C. Assertive training: A one year follow up. *Journal of Counseling Psychology*, 1975, 22, 451–452.

Gardner, R. A. *Psychotherapeutic Approaches to the Resistant Child.* New York: Aronson, 1975.

Gardner, R. A. The mutual storytelling technique in the treatment of anger inhibition problems. *Internation Journal of Child Psychotherapy*, 1971a, 1, 34–64.

Gardner, R. A. *Therapeutic Communication with Children: The Mutual Story-telling Technique.* New York: Science House, 1971b.

Geertsma, R. H. and Reivich, R. S. Repetitive self-observation by videotape playback, *Journal of Nervous and Mental Disease*, 1965, 141, 29–41.

Geocaris, K. The patient as listener. *Archives of General Psychiatry*, 1960, 2, 81–88.

Gill, M., Newman, R., and Redlich, F. *The Initial Interview in Psychiatric Practice.* New York: International Universities Press, 1954.

Goin, M. K. and Kline, F. The use of videotape in studying and teaching supervision. In Berger, M. M. (Ed.) *Videotape Techniques in Psychiatric Training and Treatment* (Second Edition). New York: Brunner/Mazel, 1978.

Goin, M. K., Kline, F. M. and Zimmerman, W. The use of videotape in teaching supervision. *Journal of Psychiatric Education*, 1978, 2(2), 189–196.

Goldfield, M. D. and Levy, R. The use of television videotape to enhance the therapeutic value of psychodrama. *American Journal of Psychiatry.* 1968, 125, 690–692.

Goldstein, M. J., Judd, L. L., Rodnick, E. H., Alkire, A. and Gould, E. A method for studying social influence and coping patterns within families of disturbed adolescents. *The Journal of Nervous and Mental Disease*, 1968, 147(3), 233–251.

Gonen, J. Y. The use of psychodrama combined with videotape playback on an inpatient floor. *Psychiatry*, 1971, 34, 198–213.

Gordon, T. *Parent Effectiveness Training*. New York: Wyden Books, 1970.

Gottheil, E., Backup, C. E. and Cornelison, F. S. Denial and self-image confrontation in a case of anorexia nervosa. *Journal of Nervous and Mental Disease*, 1969, 148, 238–250.

Greelis, M. and Kazaoka, K. The therapeutic use of edited videotapes with an exceptional child. *Academic Therapy*, 1979, 15(1), 37–44.

Greenfield, D. G. Evaluation of music therapy practicum competencies: Comparisons of self- and instructor ratings of videotapes. *Journal of Music Therapy*, 1978, 15(1), 15–20.

Greer, R. M. and Callis, R. The use of videotape models in an alcohol rehabilitation program. *Rehabilitation Counseling Bulletin*, 1975, 18(3), 154–159.

Grinnell, R. M. and Lieberman, A. Teaching the mentally retarded job interviewing skills. *Journal of Counseling Psychology*, 1977, 24(4), 332–337.

Gruenberg, P. B. and Liston, E. H. Intensive supervision of psychotherapy with videotape recording. In Berger, M. M. (Ed.) *Videotape Techniques in Psychiatric Training and Treatment* (Second Edition). New York: Brunner/Mazel, 1978.

Guerney, B. Filial therapy: Description and rationale. *Journal of Consulting Psychology*, 1964, 28, 304–310.

Gunn, R. C. A use of videotape with inpatient therapy groups. *International Journal of Group Psychotherapy*, 1978, 28(3), 365–370.

Hadden, S. B. Training. In Slavson, S. R. (Ed.) *The Fields of Group Psychotherapy*. New York: International Universities Press, Inc., 1956.

Hall, R. C. W., LeCann, A. F. and Schoolar, J. C. Amobarbital treatment of multiple personality: Use of structured video tape interviews as a basis for intensive psychotherapy. *The Journal of Nervous and Mental Disease*, 1978, 166, 666–670.

Hanser, S. B. and Furman, C. E. The effect of videotape-based feedback vs. field-based feedback on the development of applied clinical skills. *Journal of Music Therapy*, 1980, 17 (3), 103–112.

Hartlage, L. C. and Johnsen, R. P. Video playback as a rehabilitation tool with the hard core unemployed. *Rehabilitation Psychology*, 1973, 20(3), 116–120.

Hartland, J. *Medical and Dental Hypnosis*. Baltimore: Williams and Wilkins, 1971.

Hartman, W. E. and Fithian, M. A. *Treatment of Sexual Dysfunction*. Long Beach: Center for Marital and Sexual Studies, 5199 East Pacific Coast Highway, 90804, 1972.

Heckel, R. B. The television camera as co-therapist in group psychotherapy. *The Psychiatric Forum*, 1975, 5(1), 20–23.

Hector, W. Closed-circuit television for schools of nursing. *Nursing Times*, 1970, 66, 136–138.

Heidel, S., Dillon, D., Engstrom, F., Lehman, A. and Tharp, D. Medical student assessment of videocassettes in psychiatry. *Journal of Medical Education*, 1975, 50, 908–910.

Heilveil, I. Deception and pupil size. *Journal of Clinical Psychology*, 1976, 32(3), 675–676.

Heilveil, I. and Muehleman, J. T. Nonverbal clues to deception in a psychotherapy analogue. *Psychotherapy: Theory, Research and Practice.* 1981, 18(3) 329–335.

Heilveil, S. Personal communication, 1980.

Heitler, J. Preparatory techniques in initiating expressive psychotherapy with lower-class, unsophisticated patients. *Psychological Bulletin*, 1976, 83, 339–352.

Hersen, M., Eisler, R. M. and Miller, P. M. An experimental analysis of generalization in assertive training. *Behaviour Research and Therapy*, 1974, 12, 295–310.

Hogan, P. The use of videotape playback as a technique in psychotherapy. In G. D. Goldman and D. S. Milman (Eds.) *Innovations in Psychotherapy.* Springfield, Ill.: Charles C Thomas, 1972, 293.

Hogan, P. and Alger, I. The impact of V–T recording on insight in group psychotherapy. *International Journal of Group Psychotherapy*, 1969a, 19(2), 1–11.

Hogan, P. and Alger, I. Impact of videotape recording on insight in group therapy. *International Journal of Group Psychotherapy*, 1969b, 19, 158–165.

Hollander, C. and Moore, C. Rationale and guidelines for the combined use of psychodrama and videotape self-confrontation. *Group Psychotherapy and Psychodrama*, 1972, 25(3), 75–83.

Holmes, D. J. Closed circuit television in teaching psychiatry. *University of Michigan Medical Bulletin*, 1961, 27, 330–336.

Holt, D. Very special students, very special video. *Media and Methods*, 1978 (Jan), 46–48.

Holzman, P. S. On hearing and seeing oneself. *Journal of Nervous and Mental Disease*, 1969, 148, 198–209.

Horney, K. *Neurosis and human growth.* New York: Norton, 1950.

Hornsby, L. G. and Appelbaum, A. S. Parents as primary therapists: Filial therapy. In Arnold, L. E. (Ed.) *Helping Parents Help Their Children.* New York: Brunner/Mazel, 1978.

Hung, J. H. and Rosenthal, T. L. Therapeutic videotaped feedback. In Fryrear, J. L. and Fleshman, B. (Eds.) *Videotherapy in Mental Health.* Springfield, Ill.: Charles C Thomas, 1981.

Ivey, A. E. Media therapy: Educational change planning for psychiatric patients. *Journal of Counseling Psychology*, 1973, 28, 338–343.

Ivey, A. E. *Microcounseling: Innovations in Interviewing Training.* Springfield, Ill.: Charles C Thomas, 1971.

Ivey, A. E. and Authier, J. *Microcounseling: Innovations in Interviewing Counseling, Psychotherapy, and Psychoeducation.* Springfield, Ill.: Charles C Thomas, 1978.

Jankovich, R. and Miller, P. R. Response of women with primary orgasmic dysfunction to audiovisual education. *Journal of Sex and Marital Therapy,* 1978, 4, 16–19.

Kagan, N. Interpersonal process recall: Media in clinical and human interaction supervision. In Berger, M. M. (Ed.) *Videotape Techniques in Psychiatric Training and Treatment* (Second Edition). New York: Brunner/Mazel, 1978.

Kagan, N., Krathwohl, D. R. and Miller, R. Stimulated recall in therapy using videotapes: A case study. *Journal of Counseling Psychology,* 1963, 10, 237–243.

Kagan, N., Schauble, P., Resnikoff, A., Danish, S. J. and Krathwohl, D. R. Interpersonal process recall. *Journal of Nervous and Mental Disease,* 1969, 148, 365–374.

Kaplan, D. *Video in the Classroom: A Guide to Creative Television.* White Plains, NY.: Knowledge Industry Publications, Inc., 1980.

Katz, D. Videotape programming for social agencies. *Social Casework,* 1975, 56(1), 44–51.

Kaufman, G. and McElhose, R. Videotape feedback and group-splitting as facilitators of group process. *Psychotherapy: Theory, Research, and Practice,* 1973, 10(2), 167–169.

Keller, M. F. and Carlson, P. M. The use of symbolic modeling to promote social skills in preschool children with low levels of social responsiveness. *Child Development,* 1974, 45, 912–919.

Kornfield, D. S. and Kolb, L. C. The use of closed circuit TV in the teaching of psychiatry. *Journal of Nervous and Mental Disease,* 1964, 138, 452–459.

Kornhaber, R. C. and Schroeder, H. E. Importance of model similarity on extinction of avoidance behavior in children. *Journal of Consulting and Clinical Psychology,* 1975, 43, 601–607.

Krumboltz, J. D., Varenhorst, B. B. and Thoresen, C. E. Nonverbal factors in the effectiveness of models in counseling. *Journal of Counseling Psychology,* 1967, 14 (5), 412–418.

Kubie, L. S. Some aspects of the significance to psychoanalysis of the exposure of a patient to the televised audiovisual reproduction of his activities. *Journal of Nervous and Mental Disease,* 1969, 148, 301–309.

Laqueur, H. P. Multiple family therapy: Questions and answers. *Seminars in Psychiatry,* 1973, 5, 195–205.

Lautch, H. Videotape recording as an aid to behavior therapy. *British Journal of Psychiatry,* 1970, 117, 207–208.

Lazes, P. M. Community-oriented videotapes: A low-cost effective teaching tool. *International Journal of Health Education,* 1977, 20, 68–70.

Lawrence, S. B. Videotape and other therapeutic procedures with nude marathon groups. *American Psychologist*, 1969, 24, 476–479.

Lazarus, H. R. and Bienlein, D. K. Soap opera therapy. *International Journal of Group Psychotherapy*, 1967, 17, 252–256.

Lee, R. H. Video as adjunct to psychodrama and role playing. In Fryrear, J. L. and Fleshman, B. (Eds.) *Videotherapy in Mental Health.* Springfield, Ill.: Charles C Thomas, 1981.

Loeb, F. F., Jr. The microscopic film analysis of the function of a recurrent behavioral pattern in a psychotherapeutic session. *Journal of Nervous and Mental Disease*, 1968, 147, 605–618.

Long, T. J. The effects of pretraining procedures on client behavior during initial counseling interviews. *Dissertation Abstracts*, 1968, 29, 1784A.

Love, D. W., Henson, R. E., Wiese, H. J. and Parker, C. L. Controlled evaluation of videotaped interviewing for instruction of pharmacy students. *American Journal of Pharmaceutical Education*, 1979, 43(1), 3–6.

Love, A. M. and Roderick, J. A. Teacher nonverbal communication: The development and field testing of an awareness unit. *Theory Into Practice*, 1971, 10, 295–299.

Lurie, H. J. Videotape demonstrations and exercises in the psychological training of family physicians. In Berger, M. M. (Ed.) *Videotape Techniques in Psychiatric Training and Treatment* (Second Edition). New York: Brunner/Mazel, 1978.

Machen, J. and Johnson, R. Desensitization, model learning, and the dental behavior of children. *Journal of Dental Research*, 1974, 53(1), 83–87.

Mann, J. Vicarious desensitization of test anxiety through observation of videotaped treatment. *Journal of Counseling Psychology*, 1972, 19, 1–7.

Martin, G. L. and Over, H. R. Therapy by television. *Audiovisual Communication Review*, 1956, 4, 119–130.

Marvit, R. C., Lind, J. and McLaughlin, D. G. Use of videotape to induce attitude change in delinquent adolescents. *American Journal of Psychiatry*, 1974, 131, 996–999.

Mayadas, N. S. and Duehn, W. D. Stimulus-modeling (SM) videotape formats in clinical practice and research. In Fryrear, J. L. and Fleshman, B. (Eds.) *Videotherapy in Mental Health.* Springfield, Ill.: Charles C Thomas, 1981.

Mayadas, N. S. and O'Brien, D. E. The use of videotape in group psychotherapy. In Berger, M. M. (Ed.) *Videotape Techniques in Psychiatric Training and Treatment* (Second Edition). New York: Brunner/Mazel, 1978.

Mayadas, N. S. and O'Brien, D. E. The use of videotape in group psychotherapy. *Group Psychotherapy and Psychodrama*, 1973, 26, 109–119.

McMullen, S. J. Automated procedures for treatment of primary orgasmic dysfunction. *Dissertation Abstracts International*, 1976, 37(10B), 5364.

McNiff, S. Video enactment in the expressive therapies. In Fryrear, J. L. and Fleshman, B. (Eds.) *Videotherapy in Mental Health.* Springfield, Ill.: Charles C Thomas, 1981.

McNiff, S. A. and Cook, C. C. Video art therapy. *Art Psychotherapy*, 1975, 2, 55–63.

Meichenbaum, D. Examination of model characteristics in reducing avoidance behavior. *Journal of Personality and Social Psychology*, 1971, 17, 298–307.

Melamed, B. G., Hawes, R. R., Heiby, E., and Glick, J. Use of filmed modeling to reduce uncooperative behavior in children during dental treatment. *Journal of Dental Research*, 1975, 54, 797–804.

Melamed, B. and Siegel, L. Reduction of anxiety in children facing hospitalization and surgery by use of filmed modeling. *Journal of Consulting and Clinical Psychology*, 1975, 43(4), 511–521.

Metzner, R. J. Videotape self-confrontation after narcotherapy. In Berger, M. M. (Ed.) *Videotape Techniques in Psychiatric Training and Treatment* (Second Edition). New York: Brunner/Mazel, 1978.

Michel, J. and Blitstein, S. Use of videotape feedback with severely disturbed adolescents. *Child Welfare*, 1979, 58(4), 245–252.

Moore, F. J. and Chernell, E. Television as a therapeutic tool. In Berger, M. M. (Ed.) *Videotape Techniques in Psychiatric Training and Treatment* (Second Edition). New York: Brunner/Mazel, 1978.

Moore, F. J., Chernell, E. and West, M. J. Television as a therapeutic tool. *Archives of General Psychiatry*, 1965, 12, 217–222.

More, J. The use of videotape and film in sexual therapy. Paper presented at the 81st Annual Convention of the American Psychological Assn., Montreal, 1973.

Moreno, J. L. Television videotape and psychodrama. *American Journal of Psychiatry*, 1969, 125, 1453–1454.

Moreno, J. L. and Fischel, J. K. Spontaneity procedures in television broadcasting, *Sociometry*, 1942, 5(1), 7–28.

Moreno, Z. T. Psychodrama on closed and open circuit television. *Group Psychotherapy*, 1968, 21, 106–109.

Morris, R. J. and Suckerman, K. R. Therapist warmth as a factor in automated systematic desensitization. *Journal of Consulting and Clinical Psychology*, 1974, 42 (2), 244–250.

Morse, P. C. The use of video replay with disturbed children. In Berger, M. M. (Ed.) *Videotape Techniques in Psychiatric Training and Treatment* (Second Edition). New York: Brunner/Mazel, 1978.

Morse, P. C. The effects of videotaped focused feedback on competency of emotionally disturbed boys. Unpublished doctoral dissertation, Long Island University, 1976.

Mutchie, K. D., Bosso, J. A. and Higbee, M. D. Audiovisual instruction in pediatric pharmacy practice. *American Journal of Pharmaceutical Education.* 1981, 45(2), 153–155.

Nadelson, C. C., Bessuk, E. J., Hopps, C. R. and Boutelle, W. E., Jr. The use of videotape in couples therapy. *International Journal of Group Psychotherapy*, 1977, 27(2), 241–253.

Nelson, C. B. A six-year videotaped psychotherapy project with an outpatient group of schizophrenics. In Berger, M. M. (Ed.) *Videotape Techniques in Psychiatric Training and Treatment* (Second Edition). New York: Brunner/Mazel, 1978.

Noble, G., Egan, P., and McDowell, S. Changing the self-concepts of seven-year-old deprived urban children by creative drama or video feedback. *Social Behavior and Personality*, 1977, 5(1), 55–64.

O'Connor, R. Modification of social withdrawal through symbolic modeling. *Journal of Applied Behavior Analysis*, 1969, 2, 15–22.

Paredes, A., Gottheil, E., Tausig, T. N. and Cornelison, F. S., Jr. Behavioral changes as a function of repeated self-observation. *Journal of Nervous and Mental Disease*, 1969, 148(3), 287–299.

Paredes, A., Ludwig, K. D., Hassenfeld, I. N. and Cornelison, F. S., Jr. A clinical study of alcoholics using audiovisual self-image feedback. *Journal of Nervous and Mental Disease*, 1969, 148, 449–456.

Paul, N. L. Self and cross-confrontation techniques via audio- and videotape recordings in conjoint family and marital therapy. Paper presented at the American Orthopsychiatric Association, 45th Annual Meeting, Chicago, 1968.

Ramey, J. W. Teaching medical students by videotape simulation. *Journal of Medical Education*, 1968, 43, 55–59.

Rathus, S. A. Instigation of assertive behavior through videotape-mediated assertive models and directed practice. *Behavior Therapy*, 1973, 11, 57–65.

Reese, C. C. Use of video and super-8 film with drug dependent adolescents. In Fryrear, J. L. and Fleshman B. (Eds.) *Videotherapy in Mental Health*. Springfield, Ill.: Charles C Thomas, 1981.

Reivich, R. S. and Geertsma, R. H. Observational media and psychotherapy training. *Journal of Nervous and Mental Disease*, 1969, 22, 1041–1044.

Reivich, R. S. and Geertsma, R. H. Experiences with videotape self-observation by psychiatric in-patients. *Journal of the Kansas Medical Society*, 1968, 69, 39–44.

Renick, J. T. The use of films and videotapes in the treatment of sexual dysfunction. Paper presented at the 81st Annual Convention of the American Psychological Assn., Montreal, 1973.

Resnick, H. L. P., Davison, W. T., Schuyler, D. and Christopher, P. Videotape confrontation after suicide. *American Journal of Psychiatry*, 1973, 130 (4), 460–463.

Resnikoff, A., Kagan, N. and Schauble, P. G. Acceleration of psychotherapy through stimulated videotape recall. *American Journal of Psychotherapy*, 1970, 24(1), 102–111.

Robinson, C. H. The effects of observational learning on sexual behavior and attitudes in orgasmic dysfunctional women. Unpublished doctoral dissertation, University of Hawaii, 1974.

Roeske, N. C. A. The medium and the message: Development of videotapes for teaching psychiatry. *American Journal of Psychiatry*, 1979, 136 (11), 1391–1397.

Roeske, N. C. A. Videotapes as an educational experience. In Berger, M. M. (Ed.) *Videotape Techniques in Psychiatric Training and Treatment* (Second Edition). New York: Brunner/Mazel, 1978.

Rogers, C. R. The use of electrically recorded interviews in improving psychotherapeutic skills. *American Journal of Orthopsychiatry*. 1942, 12, 429.

Rosen, B. and D'Andrade, R. The psychosocial origins of achievement motivation. *Sociometry*, 1959, 22(3).

Ryan, J. Teaching and consultation by television: II. Teaching by videotape. *Mental Hospitals*, 1965, 16, 101–104.

Satir, V., Stachowiak, J. and Taschman, H. A. *Helping Families to Change*. New York: Jason Aronson, 1975.

Schaefer, H. H., Sobell, M. B., and Mills, K. C. Some sobering data on the use of self-confrontation with alcoholics. *Behavior Therapy*, 1971, 2, 28–39.

Schaefer, H. H., Sobell, M. B. and Sobell, L. C. Twelve month follow-up of hospitalized alcoholics given self-confrontation experiences by videotape. *Behavior Therapy*, 1972, 46, 36–37.

Schiff, S. B. and Reivich, R. S. Use of television as an aid to psychotherapy supervision. *Archives of General Psychiatry*, 1964, 10, 84–88.

Schlossberg, N. K. and Leibowitz, Z. B. Overview of psychological themes and content included in the five part TV series. Unpublished paper presented at the Annual Meeting of the American Psychological Assn., Los Angeles, Ca., 1981.

Schmidt, D. D. and Messner, E. The use of videotape techniques in the psychiatric training of family physicians. In Berger, M. M. (Ed.) *Videotape Techniques in Psychiatric Training and Treatment* (Second Edition). New York: Brunner/Mazel, 1978.

Schmidt, D. D. and Messner, E. The use of videotape techniques in the psychiatric training of family physicians. *Journal of Family Practice*, 1977, 5, 585.

Schnarch, D. M. Application of videotape in psychotherapy training. In Fryrear, J. L. and Fleshman, B. (Eds.) *Videotherapy in Mental Health*. Springfield, Ill.: Charles C Thomas, 1981.

Schwinghammer, T. Videotaped introductory instruction in the physical examination for clinical clerkship students. *American Journal of Pharmaceutical Education*, 1981, 45, 33–35.

Serber, M. Videotape feedback in the treatment of couples with sexual dysfunction. *Archives of Sexual Behavior*, 1974, 3, 377–380.

Serber, M. Shame aversion therapy. *Journal of Behavior Therapy and Experimental Psychiatry*, 1970, 1, 213–215.

Shipley, R. H. Extinction of conditioned fear in rats as a function of several parameters of CS exposure. *Journal of Comparative and Physiological Psychology*, 1974, 87, 699–707.

Shipley, R. H., Butt, J. H., Horwitz, B., and Farbry, J. E. Preparation for stressful medical procedure: Effect of amount of stimulus preexposure and coping style. *Journal of Consulting and Clinical Psychology*, 1978, 46, 499–507.

Shipley, R. H., Butt, J. H. and Horwitz, E. A. Preparation to reexperience a stressful medical examination: Effect of repetitious videotape exposure and coping style. *Journal of Consulting and Clinical Psychology*, 1979, 47(3), 485–492.

Shostrom, E. L. Witnessed group therapy on commercial television. *American Psychologist*, 1968, 23, 207–209.

Silk, S. The use of videotape in brief joint marital therapy. *American Journal of Psychotherapy*, 1972, 26, 417–424.

Sobell, M. B. and Sobell, L. C. Individualized behavior therapy for alcoholics. *Behavior Therapy*, 1973, 4, 49–72.

Speas, C. M. Job-seeking interview skills training: A comparison of four instructional techniques. *Journal of Counseling Psychology*, 1979, 26(5), 405–412.

Spiegel, J. P. Preface to the revised edition. In Berger, M. M. (Ed.) *Videotape Techniques in Psychiatric Training and Treatment* (Second Edition). New York: Brunner/Mazel, 1978.

Spivack, J. D. Personal process recall: Implications for psychotherapy. *Psychotherapy: Theory, Research and Practice*, 1974, 11(3), 235–238.

Stoller, F. H. Group psychotherapy on television. In Berger, M. M. (Ed.) *Videotape Techniques in Psychiatric Training and Treatment* (Second Edition). New York: Brunner/Mazel, 1978a.

Stoller, F. H. Videotape feedback in the marathon and encounter group. In Berger, M. M. (Ed.) *Videotape Techniques in Psychiatric Training and Treatment* (Second Edition). New York: Brunner/Mazel, 1978b.

Stoller, F. H. Therapeutic concepts reconsidered in light of videotape experience. *Comparative Group Studies*, 1970, 1, 5–17.

Stoller, F. H. Videotape feedback in the group setting. *Journal of Nervous and Mental Disease*, 1969, 148, 457–466.

Stoller, F. H. Accelerated interaction: A time-limited approach based on the brief intensive group. *International Journal of Group Psychotherapy*, 1968a, 18, 220–258.

Stoller, F. H. Use of videotape (focused feedback) in group counseling and group therapy. *Journal of Research and Development in Education*, 1968b, 1, 30–44.

Stoller, F. H. Focused feedback with videotape: Extending the group's functions. In G. M. Gazda (Ed.) *Innovations to Group Therapy and Counseling*, Springfield, Ill.: Charles C Thomas, 1968c.

Stoller, F. H. Group psychotherapy on television. An innovation with hospitalized patients. *American Psychologist*, 1967a, 22, 158–162.

Stoller, F. H. The long weekend. *Psychology Today*, 1967b, 1, 28–33.

Stuart, R. B. *Helping Couples Change*. New York: The Guilford Press, 1980a.

Stuart, R. B. *Getting Marriage Therapy Off on the Right Foot*. New York: BMA/Guilford, 1980b.

Suess, J. F. Teaching psychodiagnosis and observation by self-instructional programmed videotapes. *Journal of Medical Education*, 1973, 48, 676–683.

Suess, J. F. Teaching clinical psychiatry with closed circuit television and videotape. *Journal of Medical Education*, 1966, 41, 483–488.

Tardiff, K. A videotape technique for measuring clinical skills: Three years of experience. *Journal of Medical Education*, 1981, 56(3), 187–191.

Thelen, M. H., Fry, E. A., Dollinger, S. J. and Paul, S. J. Use of videotaped models to improve the interpersonal adjustment to delinquents. *Journal of Consulting and Clinical Psychology*, 1976, 44, 492.

Thelen, M. H., Fry, R. A., Fehrenbach, P. A. and Frautschi, N. M. Developments in therapeutic videotape and film modeling. In Fryrear, J. L. and Fleshman, B. (Eds.) *Videotherapy in Mental Health*. Springfield, Ill.: Charles C Thomas, 1981.

Thelen, M. H., Fry, R. A., Fehrenbach, P. A. and Frautschi, N. M. Therapeutic videotape and film modeling: A review. *Psychological Bulletin*, 1979, 86(4), 701–720.

Thomas, G. M. Using videotaped modeling to increase attending behavior. *Elementary School Guidance and Counseling*, 1974, 9, 35–40.

Travis, R. L. The language of the body. *Media and Methods*, 1977 (Sept.), 106–110.

Trethowan, W. H. Teaching psychiatry with closed-circuit television. *British Journal of Psychiatry*, 1968, 114, 517–522.

Truax, C. and Wargo, D. Effects of vicarious therapy pretraining and alternate sessions on outcome of group psychotherapy with outpatients. *Journal of Consulting and Clinical Psychology*, 1969, 33, 509–521.

Ulett, F. A., Akpinar, S. and Itil, T. M. Hypnosis by videotape. *International Journal of Clinical and Experimental Hypnosis*, 1972, 20, 46–51.

Vandervoort, H. E. and Blank, J. E. A sex counseling program in a university medical center. *The Counseling Psychologist*, 1975, 5, 64–67.

Van Zoost, B. Premarital communication skills education with university students. *Family Coordinator*, 1973, 22, 187–191.

Vernon, D. T. A. Use of modeling to modify children's responses to a natural, potentially stressful situation. *Journal of Applied Psychology*, 1973, 58(3), 351–356.

Vernon, D. T. A. and Bailey, W. The use of motion pictures in the psychological preparation of children for induction of anesthesia. *Anesthesiology*, 1974, 40, 68–72.

Vernon, D. T. A., Foley, J. M. Sipowicz, R. R. and Schulman, J. L. *The Psychological Responses of Children to Hospitalization and Illness*. Springfield, Ill.: Charles C Thomas, 1965.

Vernon, D. T. A., Schulman, J. L. and Foley, J. M. Changes in children's behavior after hospitalization. *American Journal of the Diseases of Children*, 1966, 3, 581–593.

Vogler, R. E. and Caddy, G. R. Treatment and prevention of alcoholism: The moderation approach. Proceedings of the Eighty-second Annual Convention of the American Psychological Association, 1973, 931–932.

Vogler, R. E., Weissbach, T. A. and Compton, J. V. Learning techniques for alcohol abuse. *Behavior Research and Therapy*, 1977, 15(1), 31–38.

Wachtel, A. B., Stein, A. and Baldinger, M. Dynamic implications of videotape recording and playback in analytic group psychotherapy. *International Journal of Group Psychotherapy*, 1979, 29, 67–85.

Walkenshaw, M. R. An investigation into the possible therapeutic usefulness of videotape self-confrontation. *Dissertation Abstracts International*, 1973, 33(12-A), 6759.

Watters, W. W., Elder, P., Smith, S. L. and Cleghorn, J. Psychotherapy supervision: A videotape technique. *Canadian Psychiatry Association Journal*, 1971, 16, 367–368.

Waxer, P. H. Short-term group psychotherapy: Some principles and techniques. *International Journal of Group Psychotherapy*, 1977, 7, 33–41.

Waxer, P. H. Therapist training in nonverbal communication. II. Nonverbal cues for depression. *Journal of Clinical Psychology*, 1974, 30, 215–218.

Weir, W. D. Evaluating psychiatric learning through videotaped patient interviews. In Berger, M. M. (Ed.) *Videotape Techniques in Psychiatric Training and Treatment* (Second Edition). New York: Brunner/Mazel, 1978.

Weir, W. D. Clinical psychiatry videotest. *Biomedical Communications*. 1975, 3(5), 17, 27.

Whitaker, C. The use of videotape in family therapy with special relation to the therapeutic impasse. In Berger, M. M. (Ed.) *Videotape Techniques in Psychiatric Training and Treatment* (Second Edition). New York: Brunner/Mazel, 1978.

Whitehorn, J. C. Attempts to teach principles of psychiatric interviewing. *Southern Medical Journal*, 1941, 34, 1130–1136.

Wicklund, R. A. Objective self-awareness. In L. Berkowitz (Ed.) *Advances in Experimental Social Psychology* (Vol. 8). New York: Academic Press, 1975.

Wilmer, H. A. Use of the television monologue with adolescent psychiatric patients. *American Journal of Psychiatry*. 1970, 126, 1760–1766.

Wilmer, H. A. Innovative uses of videotape on a psychiatric ward. *Hospital and Community Psychiatry*, 1968, 19(5), 21–25.

Wilmer, H. A. Practical and theoretical aspects of videotape supervision in psychiatry. *Journal of Nervous and Mental Disease*, 1967, 145, 123–130.

Wincze, J. P. and Caird, W. K. The effects of systematic desensitization and video desensitization in the treatment of essential sexual dysfunction in women. *Behavior Therapy*, 1976, 7, 335–342.

Wolpe, J. *The Practice of Behavior Therapy*. New York: Pergamon Press, 1969.

Woody, R. H. Clinical suggestion in videotaped psychotherapy: A research progress report. *American Journal of Clinical Hypnosis*, 1971, 14, 32–37.

Woody, R. H. Clinical suggestion and the videotaped vicarious desensitization method. *American Journal of Clinical Hypnosis*, 1969, 11(4), 239–244.

Woody, R. H. and Schauble, P. G. Videotaped vicarious desensitization. *Journal of Nervous and Mental Disease*, 1969b, 148, 281–286.

Woody, R. H., Krathwohl, D. R., Kagan, N. and Farquhar, W. W. Stimulated recall in psychotherapy using hypnosis and videotape. *American Journal of Clinical Hypnosis*, 1965, 7(3), 234–241.

Woody, R. H. and Schauble, P. G. Desensitization of fear by videotapes. *Journal of Clinical Psychology*, 1969a, 25, 102–103.

Woody, R. H. and Schauble, P. G. Videotaped vicarious desensitization. *Journal of Nervous and Mental Disease*, 1969b, 148, 281–286.

Wroblewski, P. F., Jacob, T. and Rehm, L. P. The contribution of relaxation to symbolic modeling in the modification of dental fears. *Behavior Research and Therapy*, 1977, 15, 113–115.

# Index

# VIDEOTAPES AVAILABLE FROM TAVISTOCK

## A CONVERSATIONAL MODEL OF PSYCHOTHERAPY: A TEACHING METHOD
### Robert Hobson & Frank Margison

In this three-tape video package Robert Hobson and Frank Margison demonstrate the model's use of direct statements rather than questions; a negotiating style; recognition of cues; staying with and focusing on feelings; making links inside and outside the session; and the use of metaphorical language.

## HANDLING DIFFICULT QUESTIONS
### Peter Maguire

This tape emphasizes the essential but often neglected communication skills that hospital professionals must draw on when caring for the emotional and physical well-being of cancer patients.

## BREAKING BAD NEWS
### David Goldberg

The tape deals with the way bad news is broken to the relatives of patients who are suffering from fatal illnesses.

## KEY ELEMENTS IN THE HELPING INTERVIEW
### Malcolm J. Brown

What are the key elements of a successful interview? Malcolm Brown looks at the ways of handling an intake interview with a young mother who seems to have been deserted by her husband.

## DEPRESSION: UNDERSTANDING AND HELPING
### Malcolm J. Brown

From an introduction covering the signs of depression, how help might be given, and the requirements of the 1983 Mental Health Act, Malcolm Brown presents and comments on three role-played interactions: reactive depression, agitated depression, and catatonic depression.

## UNDERSTANDING AND HANDLING AGGRESSION
### Malcolm J. Brown

Through several role-played interviews and interactions, and with reference to the 1983 Mental Health Act, Malcolm Brown suggests ways of defusing difficult encounters and helping the client.